A nutritionist's
guide to over
180 healthy juice
and smoothie
recipes

THE
DAILY
BOOST

NICOLA DESCHAMPS

hamlyn

hamlyn

First published in Great Britain in 2024
by Hamlyn, an imprint of
Octopus Publishing Group Ltd,
Carmelite House,
50 Victoria Embankment,
London EC4Y 0DZ
www.octopusbooks.co.uk

An Hachette UK Company
www.hachette.co.uk

Some of this material previously
appeared in *Hamlyn All Colour
Cookbook: 200 Juices & Smoothies,
Hamlyn All Colour Cookbook: Juice
Diet Recipes* by Joy Skipper.

Distributed in the US by Hachette
Book Group, 1290 Avenue of the
Americas, 4th and 5th Floors,
New York NY 10104

Distributed in Canada by Canadian
Manda Group, 664 Annette Street,
Toronto, Ontario, Canada M6S 2C8

ISBN 978-0-600-63886-5

A CIP catalogue record for this book is
available from the British Library.
Printed and bound in China.

10 9 8 7 6 5 4 3 2 1

Commissioning Editor: Louisa
Johnson
Photographers: Vanessa Davies,
Janine Hosegood, Lis Parsons,
Gareth Sambridge
Art director: Jaz Bahra
Project Editor: Vicky Orchard
Deputy Picture Manager: Jennifer Veal
Production Manager: Caroline Alberti

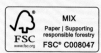

MIX
Paper | Supporting
responsible forestry
FSC
www.fsc.org   FSC® C008047

Picture credits
Vanessa Davies 36, 51, 101, 107; Janine
Hosegood 110, 114; Lis Parsons 24, 25,
27, 28, 30, 31, 32, 33, 34, 35, 37, 38, 39, 40,
41, 42, 43, 44, 45, 47, 48, 49, 50, 52, 53,
54, 55, 56, 57, 59, 60, 61, 62, 63, 64, 65,
66, 67, 68, 69, 70, 71, 72, 73, 74, 75, 76, 77,
78, 79, 80, 81, 82, 83, 84, 85, 86, 87, 88,
89, 90, 91, 92, 93, 94, 95, 96, 97, 98, 99,
100, 102, 103, 104, 105, 106, 108, 109, 111,
112, 113, 115, 116, 118, 119, 120, 121, 122, 123;
Gareth Sambidge 26, 29, 46, 58, 117.

Cookery notes
Standard level spoon measurement
are used in all recipes.
1 tablespoon - one 15 ml spoon
1 teaspoon - one 5 ml spoon

200 ml (7 fl oz) makes one average
serving

Both imperial and metric
measurements have been given in all
recipes. Use one set of measurements
only and not a mixture of both.

Pepper should be freshly ground black
pepper unless otherwise stated.

CONTENTS

INTRODUCTION

Making a splash

Everyone wants to look and feel their best from the inside out, and nutrition can help. Drinking fresh, raw juices and smoothies regularly will put you on the path to good health.

Choose from over 180 delicious drinks that can provide your body with nourishing nutrients to boost your health. The recipes are simple and use ingredients found in most supermarkets. Weekly recipe planners will help inspire and guide you and save you time and money. Highlighted in every recipe is a nutrient that benefits a specific part of the body.

What is the difference between a juice and a smoothie?

The main difference is how these drinks are made – a juicer is used to make juices, and a blender for smoothies. Juice is the liquid extracted from fruits or vegetables, whereas a smoothie is a blend of whole fruits, vegetables, and sometimes other ingredients. Juice is a concentrated source of liquid nutrients (including fruit sugars) with little to no fibre left as the pulp is removed. A smoothie includes everything, and nothing is removed, making it thicker and more dense in texture than a thin, easier-to-digest liquid. Besides fruits and vegetables, other ingredients like nuts or seeds are typically added to smoothies. Nutritional powders, such as wheatgrass and extra virgin plant oils, are sometimes added to a juice. Both drinks offer a quick and convenient way of hitting the recommended five-a-day fruit and vegetable target.

What are the health benefits of drinking juices and smoothies?

Numerous! Whether you juice or blend, both options provide a convenient way to get a daily dose of nutrients and are welcome additions to a balanced diet. You know what you're getting with home-produced juices and smoothies – they are fresh, additive-free, unpasteurized, have no added sugars, and are not made from concentrates. Plus, you get to make drinks using your favourite ingredients.

Eating a well-balanced, varied and nutritious diet gives your body the nutrients it needs to function at its best. Fruits and vegetables are packed with vitamins, minerals, antioxidants, enzymes and powerful phytonutrients (plant chemicals) that can enhance health and offer protection from disease. Enjoying juices and smoothies as part of your diet can strengthen immune defences, promote gut health, boost energy, support detoxification, aid weight management, and leave you feeling revitalized.

Plant-based foods contain various vitamins, minerals and protective components that support the immune system. Fibre-rich smoothies fuel beneficial gut bacteria that help support good digestion and are known to play an important role in the immune system. Vitamins and minerals, such as vitamin C and zinc, help heal wounds and fight infection, while phytonutrients have been shown to have antibacterial, antifungal and antiviral properties. Fruits and vegetables are rich in antioxidants, which can beneficially influence processes responsible for inflammation in the body.

When you experience stress, your brain sends signals to your gut that can lead to digestive issues and inflammation. Enjoying fresh homemade juices and smoothies can be beneficial because they contain high levels of antioxidants that might help maintain and protect your gut while helping reduce inflammation. Certain foods may help reduce cortisol levels and boost serotonin, a calming brain chemical. Being extra busy can lead to feeling stressed and eating healthily becomes more challenging. Nutrient-rich smoothies are perfect standbys when there's no time to prepare healthy meals or if you're on the go and tempted to stop for an unhealthy takeaway high in fat and salt.

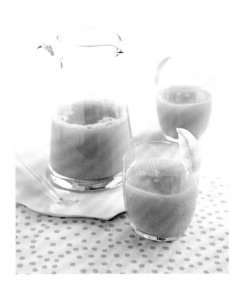

Modern life can be hectic, so it is important to have enough energy to last the day. A juice or smoothie with good calories and nutrients that stimulate energy production can help you stay on top of your game. A vitamin-laden, energy-boosting juice will help improve focus and memory. Juices deliver easily absorbed concentrated amounts of natural sugars and essential nutrients, making them a quick energy source and ideal as a light, pre-workout snack. Using water-rich fruits and vegetables in your drinks offers a natural way to help you keep hydrated and replace lost minerals during exercise. Protein-rich smoothies containing nut butter or yogurt are great recovery boosters, providing the body with the building blocks needed to repair and refuel tired muscles post-exercise.

The body is hardwired to clean itself, with a built-in system designed to remove unwanted toxins. However, increasing exposure to environmental pollutants inside and outside our homes can impact our health and wellbeing. Cleansing juices and smoothies can support the body's natural cleansing system by supporting the organs responsible for removing waste and toxins from the body – colon, kidneys, liver, lungs and skin. Some natural foods help stimulate the kidneys to remove toxins from the blood or urine and support the liver to break down harmful substances. Others stimulate the bowel, helping to eliminate waste through the large intestine.

For those watching their weight, too busy to eat, or feeling unwell, smoothies rich in proteins and fibre can provide a filling meal in a glass. Fibre slows digestion, helps balance blood sugars, makes you feel full, and reduces cravings, which can aid weight loss. Juices and smoothies low in calories and high in antioxidants are helpful for those recovering from illness who need fuel that nourishes and heals but requires little effort to digest.

Neither juices nor smoothies should replace whole fruits and vegetables in your diet, but both drinks can significantly increase your daily fruit and vegetable intake, making them invaluable additions to a balanced whole foods diet that focuses on plants, whole grains, nuts, legumes and seeds. Not only are homemade juices and smoothies delicious, but they also offer more bang for your buck! Compared to many convenience foods and drinks, fresh fruits and vegetables are budget-friendly and are nutrient-rich and good for your health.

What is the best equipment to use to make juices and smoothies?

This largely depends on budget. The most common types of juicers are masticating (slow) and centrifugal (fast). A fast juicer uses a flat cutting blade that pushes the juice through a spinning basket, separating the pulp. The high speed of the blade generates noise plus heat, which, together with oxidation, can lead to some nutrient loss. However, these juicers are considered good entry-level buys for starters on a tight budget.

The best juicer for preserving valuable nutrients is a masticating juicer, which uses an auger to slowly crush and squeeze out the maximum amount of juice and separate the pulp. Although more

expensive, the masticating juicer offers a comparably higher juice yield, and the slower extraction process makes it quieter.

Making juices without a juicer is possible by using a high-speed electric blender. After blending, all ingredients must be strained through a nut milk bag or muslin cloth to remove the pulp. Juice pulp can be used to thicken stews and soups, flavour dips or added to compost.

Blenders have a motorized base and a jug and usually have one propeller-like blade that pulverizes foods. Jug blenders or smoothie makers are good options and vary in size and function. Smoothie makers are smaller and typically come with lids, allowing you to drink on-the-go. A stick blender is a low-cost option but may take a bit longer to handle tough-to-break-down ingredients.

What are the healthiest ingredients to include in your juices and smoothies?

All fruits and vegetables have beneficial properties; there is no one most healthy fruit or vegetable. Having a variety of both every day will help improve your health and wellbeing. Equally important is finding recipes you love. When you enjoy what you're drinking, making juices and smoothies part of your regular routine will become much easier. A tasty juice formula usually includes something juice-rich, sweet, sharp and earthy, including a spice or herb as an optional extra.

Here are some examples:

Sweet:
apples, carrots, mangoes, beetroots, bananas, blueberries, melons, pineapples, kiwifruit, grapes, tomatoes, bell peppers, parsnips

Sharp:
oranges, lemons, limes, grapefruits, cranberries, raspberries, redcurrants

Juicy:
apples, pears, melons, pineapples, cucumber, celery, tomatoes, mangoes

Earthy:
beetroots, carrots, parsnips, fennel, spinach, apricots

Herbs:
parsley, coriander, mint

Spices:
ginger, cinnamon, chilli (a little), garlic (a little, too)

Both juices and smoothies are a great way to pack in even more nutrients with the addition of extra virgin plant oils, nuts, seeds and nutrition powders, such as wheatgrass and spices or herbs. Try protein-rich ingredients like pea protein, chia seeds or flaxseeds for smoothies. There is a huge variety to choose from, and each one offers its own benefits. For example, a few drops of extra virgin olive oil in your juice will help with the absorption of fat-soluble nutrients like vitamins A, D, E and K. Plus, olive oil is rich in monounsaturated fatty acids, which research has shown to reduce the risk of heart disease. A spoonful of nut butter in your smoothie boosts its protein content, provides a great energy source and includes beneficial fats such as omega 3 and 6.

As with any food, it's best to choose those without unwanted extras such as pesticides, herbicides, fungicides, hormones, etc. Wash and scrub all fresh produce and choose unwaxed citrus fruit. If possible, choose organic and shop locally and seasonally. How a plant is grown, processed and stored can affect its nutrient content. Every country has their own food standards, processes and regulations.

How can you keep your fruits and vegetables fresher for longer?
Fresh fruits and vegetables have a shelf life. Once they've been harvested, the clock starts ticking. However, there are a few top tips that can help preserve produce for longer.

Buy local, at a farmers' market, farm shop, or from a vegetable box scheme. The fewer the steps from field to fork, the better. Fruits and vegetables grown locally are generally fresher and tastier, as they're harvested at the right time and don't spend days or weeks on the road or being processed and handled.

Remove plant tops or leaves
Plant tops absorb moisture from fruit or vegetables, drying them out. Leafy green tops, such as those on carrots, should be removed and stored separately (and eaten if edible).

Wash and scrub
Washing your fresh produce helps remove unwanted extras like dirt, unseen bacteria and pesticides, improving the safety and quality of your fruits and vegetables and extending their shelf life.

Dry excess moisture
Make sure your fruits and vegetables are thoroughly dry before storing them. Removing moisture will help prevent bacteria from growing, which can cause rotting and contamination.

Bag it
Fresh produce can stay fresh for a longer period if it is sealed and protected from the cold conditions in the refrigerator and freezer. Place produce in containers, zip-top bags, or pouches, or wrap them, especially delicate herbs, in kitchen paper. Avoid pushing produce to the back of the refrigerator, where it may get too cold and icy.

Eat it
The softer the produce gets, the quicker it needs to be used. Planning ahead is key to avoiding waste, saving money and reducing your carbon footprint.

Freeze it
If you have a surplus of produce or think you won't have time to use it, then wash, dry and store it in the freezer. Herbs can be chopped, mixed with extra virgin olive oil, and stored in ice-cube trays. Once frozen, they can be placed into freezer bags and used as needed.

Ethylene gas
It is important to store fruits and vegetables that produce ethylene gas, such as bananas, separately from those that are sensitive to it, as ethylene can speed up the ripening process.

No heat
Fresh produce should be stored away from heated appliances like radiators, as high temperatures can speed up ripening. It should also be stored out of the way of direct sunlight.

Drinking juices and smoothies immediately is best since nutrients decrease over time, making the drink less nutritious. If this is not possible, store your juice or smoothie in an airtight glass container, refrigerate and consume within 24 hours.

Cost-cutting ingredient alternatives

- avoid pre-washed, pre-cut and ready-to-eat fruit and vegetables, which come with a premium price

- aim to buy fresh produce in its natural state. Try picking up a whole mango instead of a pre-cut mango in a plastic pot, or opt for a head of broccoli instead of a bag of florets

- buy imperfect produce! Supermarkets prefer produce that is consistent in shape and size, but irregularly shaped fruits and vegetables are just as nutritious

- shop at your local farmers' market

- buy discounted fruits and vegetables and freeze them if you can't use them straight away

- pick or grow your own fruits and vegetables and freeze any surplus

- make your own nut butters and plant milks using a food processor or blender

- partner with friends to buy seeds and nuts in bulk, then store them in airtight containers

- frozen fruit and vegetables are usually cheaper than fresh ones. Flash-frozen just a few hours after picking, the nutrient profiles of commercially frozen fruit and vegetables are similar to fresh

- opt for canned fruit in natural fruit juice rather than syrup

- choose fruits in season as they're cheaper. Often, a glut of produce can mean price reductions. For example, cranberries are seasonal and appear in supermarkets during Christmas. Buy and freeze them to use later in the year

- freeze-dried fruits offer a longer shelf life

Is supplementation necessary?

Dietary supplements are concentrated nutrients derived from either plant or animal sources. They contain specific nutrients and come in different forms, such as tablets, powders, liquids and capsules. These supplements are either artificially created or extracted from food sources.

We all know that our diet has a huge impact on our physical and mental health and wellbeing. That's why many of us want to take charge of our own health, either to achieve optimal health or reduce the risk of illness or chronic disease. Recent nutritional research has highlighted the power of plant-based foods and their potential to heal and help us stay healthy. As a result, there has been a surge in the development of nutritional powders and dietary supplements.

Typically, nutrients are better absorbed from foods than supplements. Some supplements can interact with one another and, if taken in excess, can cause unpleasant symptoms and, in some cases, lead to toxic build-up. Generally, water-soluble vitamins are less likely to cause problems as any excess is excreted in your urine. In moderate amounts, a quality protein powder or green powder, such as spirulina or wheatgrass, can provide a nutritional boost to juices and smoothies.

Most healthcare professionals agree that a varied, balanced and whole food diet provides most people with the necessary nutrients to maintain health. However, some supplements, such as vitamins D, B12, B9 (folate), and iron, are recommended for certain groups of people, including:

- vegetarians, vegans and people on special diets
- pregnant women or those wanting to conceive
- elderly or housebound people
- people who get little or no sun exposure, those with darker skin and children under five years of age
- individuals with specific diseases that impact nutrient absorption, such as inflammatory bowel disease

For more specific needs or if you're concerned about deficiency, it is advisable to seek professional guidance from a doctor, dietician or registered nutritionist.

The last drop

No juice or smoothie can make you healthy, but they can help you sip your way to 'five-a-day'! Learning about the nutritional properties of different fruits and vegetables empowers you to make informed choices. Investing in your health is one of the most valuable things you can do for yourself. Your body will thank you in the long run. When it comes to developing good dietary habits, there are no shortcuts or quick fixes. Consistency is key to forming new healthy habits, together with learning to love what is good for you. Experiencing positive change and feeling and seeing the benefits of nourishing your body is so rewarding.

In every recipe, I've highlighted a nutrient that benefits a specific part of the body, as illustrated by the icons opposite. Remember, many recipes contain multiple health-giving ingredients – this guide is just here to help focus your health goals!

KEY

SKIN

WEIGHT

HEART

GUT

BONE

BRAIN

MUSCLE

**IMMUNE
SYSTEM**

EYES

DETOX

**NERVOUS
SYSTEM**

ENERGY

REPRODUCTION

**ENDOCRINE
SYSTEM**

URINARY

WEEK 1
SMOOTHIE RECIPES

MONDAY
energizer smoothie

TUESDAY
cucumber, lemon & mint smoothie

WEDNESDAY
banana & tahini smoothie

THURSDAY
orange, mango & strawberry smoothie

FRIDAY
perfect passion smoothie

SATURDAY
banana, orange & mango smoothie

SUNDAY
tropical fruit smoothie

SHOPPING LIST

Fresh Fruit / Veg
1 beetroot, about 200 g (7 oz)
3 ripe bananas
125 g (4 oz) strawberries
100 g (3½ oz) blackberries
5 passion fruit
5 ripe mangoes
3–4 fresh mint leaves
250 g (8 oz) cucumber
1 lemon
1 lime
pineapple chunks (optional)
orange slices (optional)

Refrigerator / Freezer
300 ml (½ pint) pineapple juice
500 ml (17 fl oz) orange juice
375 ml (13 fl oz) natural yogurt
500 ml (17 fl oz) semi-skimmed
    milk
500 ml (17 fl oz) almond milk
fromage frais

Storecupboard
6 stoned dates
rolled oats
maca powder
ground flaxseed
tahini paste

WEEK 1
JUICE RECIPES

MONDAY
blueberry, apple & ginger juice

TUESDAY
carrot, chicory & celery juice

WEDNESDAY
healing green juice

THURSDAY
virgin piña colada juice

FRIDAY
carrot, beetroot & sweet potato juice

SATURDAY
kickstart juice

SUNDAY
healthy green punch

SHOPPING LIST

Fresh Fruit / Veg
250 g (8 oz) blueberries
125 g (4 oz) grapefruit
550 g (15 oz) apples
500 g (17 oz) carrots
250 g (8 oz) celery
125 g (4 oz) chicory
40 g (1½ oz) kale
30 g (1¼ oz) spinach
1 Little Gem lettuce, about 140 g
    (4½ oz)
1 cucumber, about 175 g (6 oz)
400 g (13 oz) pineapple
175 g (6 oz) sweet potato
100 g (3½ oz) beetroot
125 g (4 oz) fennel
6 lemons
1 garlic clove
100 g (3½ oz) alfalfa sprouts
fresh horseradish root
fresh root ginger
15 g (½ oz) parsley

Refrigerator / Freezer
200 ml (7 fl oz) coconut water

Storecupboard
spirulina powder
hemp seed oil

WEEK 2
SMOOTHIE RECIPES

MONDAY
mango, coconut & lime lassi

TUESDAY
mango, apple & blackcurrant smoothie

WEDNESDAY
red pepper & tomato smoothie

THURSDAY
cranberry & apple smoothie

FRIDAY
nutty recovery smoothie

SATURDAY
almond milk & banana smoothie

SUNDAY
pineapple, parsnip & carrot smoothie

SHOPPING LIST

Fresh Fruit / Veg
4 large ripe mangoes
1 lime
1 orange
200 g (7 oz) blackcurrants
5 bananas
4 medjool dates
50 g (2 oz) red pepper
50 g (2 oz) cucumber
30 g (1¼ oz) spring onion
splash of lemon juice
250 g (8 oz) apple
250 g (8 oz) pineapple
100 g (3½ oz) parsnip
100 g (3½ oz) carrot

Refrigerator / Freezer
400 ml (14 fl oz) natural yogurt
100 ml (3½ fl oz) apple juice
100 ml (3½ fl oz) tomato juice
600 ml (1 pint) almond milk
75 ml (3 fl oz) soya milk
2 tablespoons mango sorbet
100 g (3½ oz) frozen cranberries

Storecupboard
clear honey
400 ml (14 fl oz) coconut milk
hot pepper sauce
Worcestershire sauce
peanut butter
¼ teaspoon ground cinnamon
grated nutmeg, to sprinkle

WEEK 2
JUICE RECIPES

MONDAY
orange, apple & pear juice

TUESDAY
spinach, tomato & broccoli juice

WEDNESDAY
apple, pineapple & melon juice

THURSDAY
watermelon cooler

FRIDAY
beet treat juice

SATURDAY
blackberry, apple & celeriac juice

SUNDAY
lettuce & kiwifruit juice

SHOPPING LIST

Fresh Fruit / Veg
3 oranges
2 red apples
3 green apples
1 pear
2 tomatoes
1 galia melon
1 pineapple
100 g (3½ oz) watermelon
100 g (3½ oz) strawberries
100 g (3½ oz) kiwifruit
2 beetroots
100 g (3½ oz) red cabbage
100 g (3½ oz) celeriac
1 celery stick (optional)
150 g (5 oz) spinach
150 g (5 oz) broccoli
200 g (7 oz) lettuce
mint or tarragon leaves

Refrigerator / Freezer
100 g (3½ oz) frozen blackberries

Storecupboard
clear honey (optional)

WEEK 3
SMOOTHIE RECIPES

MONDAY
strawberry & soya smoothie

TUESDAY
blueberry & mint smoothie

WEDNESDAY
mango & mint sherbet

THURSDAY
peach & orange smoothie

FRIDAY
peach & tofu smoothie

SATURDAY
mandarin & lychee frappé

SUNDAY
heavenly hemp smoothie

SHOPPING LIST

Fresh Fruit / Veg
100 g (3½ oz) fresh or frozen
    strawberries
2 kiwifruit
3 ripe mangoes
100 g (3½ oz) peach
1 papaya, about 250 g (8 oz)
1 apricot, about 75 g (3 oz)
1 lime, plus extra to decorate
small bunch of mint
lemon juice

Refrigerator / Freezer
100 g (3½ oz) tofu
150 ml (¼ pint) natural yogurt, plus
    extra to serve
200 ml (7 fl oz) orange juice
350 ml (12 fl oz) soya milk
400 ml (14 fl oz) hemp milk
50 g (2 oz) vanilla coconut ice cream
100 g (3½ oz) frozen blueberries

Storecupboard
400 g (13 oz) can peaches in
    natural juice
100 g (3½ oz) mandarin oranges,
    canned in natural juice
50 g (2 oz) lychees, canned in
    natural juice
few drops of natural almond essence
clear honey (optional)
1 teaspoon chia oil
¼ teaspoon ground cinnamon
25 g (1 oz) flaked almonds (optional)

WEEK 3
JUICE RECIPES

MONDAY
orange & cranberry juice

TUESDAY
tomato, orange & celery juice

WEDNESDAY
strawberry, redcurrant & orange juice

THURSDAY
forest fruits juice

FRIDAY
broccoli, spinach & apple juice

SATURDAY
citrus green juice

SUNDAY
melon, carrot & ginger juice

SHOPPING LIST

Fresh Fruit / Veg
5 carrots
5 oranges
2 celery sticks
4 tomatoes
3 apples
100 g (3½ oz) strawberries
75 g (3 oz) redcurrants
225 g (7½ oz) cranberries
200 g (7 oz) blackberries
100 g (3½ oz) blueberries
1 grapefruit, about 275 g (9 oz)
250 g (8 oz) cantaloupe melon
150 g (5 oz) broccoli
150 g (5 oz) spinach
2 limes
1 cm (½ inch) piece fresh
    root ginger

Storecupboard
clear honey (optional)
agave syrup
wheatgrass powder

WEEK 4
SMOOTHIE RECIPES

MONDAY
rhubarb smoothie

TUESDAY
mango, pineapple & lime smoothie

WEDNESDAY
raspberry, kiwifruit & grapefruit smoothie

THURSDAY
cherry & chocolate smoothie

FRIDAY
raspberry & blueberry smoothie

SATURDAY
breakfast nut smoothie

SUNDAY
nectarine & raspberry yogurt smoothie

SHOPPING LIST

Fresh Fruit / Veg
100 g (3½ oz) stewed rhubarb
3 nectarines
1 ripe mango
1 lime
1 banana
2 oranges
425 g (14 oz) raspberries
200 g (7 oz) blueberries
150 g (5 oz) grapefruit
175 g (6 oz) pineapple
50 g (2 oz) kiwifruit

Refrigerator / Freezer
250 ml (8 fl oz) natural yogurt
4 tablespoons Greek yogurt
300 ml (½ pint) pineapple juice
200 ml (7 fl oz) apple juice
400 ml (14 fl oz) skimmed milk
50 g (2 oz) frozen raspberries
50 g (2 oz) frozen cranberries

Storecupboard
muesli
cashew nuts
ground cinnamon
vanilla extract
clear honey
wheatgerm (optional)

WEEK 4
JUICE RECIPES

MONDAY

fabulous fennel juice

TUESDAY

tomato, red pepper & papaya juice

WEDNESDAY

melon, carrot & ginger juice

THURSDAY

carrot, cabbage & apple juice

FRIDAY

pear, celery & ginger juice

SATURDAY

fennel & camomile juice

SUNDAY

tomato, carrot & ginger juice

SHOPPING LIST

Fresh Fruit / Veg

1 large tomato + 300 g
    (10 oz) tomatoes
1 lime
1 lemon
1 garlic clove
1 orange (optional)
2 fennel bulbs, about
    300 g (10 oz)
4 apples, about 325 g
    (11 oz)
5 carrots, about 625 g (1¼ lb)
100 g (3½ oz) red pepper
100 g (3½ oz) pear
125 g (4 oz) papaya
125 g (4 oz) red cabbage
150 g (5 oz) celery
250 g (8 oz) cantaloupe melon
fresh root ginger
fresh horseradish

Refrigerator / Freezer

100 ml (3½ fl oz) chilled
    camomile tea

Storecupboard

grated nutmeg

WEIGHT MANAGEMENT
SMOOTHIE RECIPES

MONDAY
banana & pineapple smoothie
BENEFIT: reduces hunger

TUESDAY
creamy green smoothie
BENEFIT: reduces belly fat

WEDNESDAY
kiwifruit, mango & raspberry smoothie
BENEFIT: blood sugar balance

THURSDAY
banana & maple syrup smoothie
BENEFIT: low GI

FRIDAY
banana & chocolate smoothie
BENEFIT: calming*
*Low magnesium levels have been linked to low
mood, which may lead to poor food choices.*

SATURDAY
cherry & chocolate smoothie
BENEFIT: lowers uric acid*
*Obese patients face a higher risk of
developing gout.*

SUNDAY
melon, mint & berry smoothie
BENEFIT: hydrating*
*Well-hydrated individuals are less likely
to snack.*

SHOPPING LIST

Fresh Fruit / Veg
4 bananas
2 ripe mangoes
1 avocado
1 lime
2 celery sticks
3 kiwifruit
1 garlic clove
30 g (1¼ oz) spinach
25 g (1 oz) parsley
150 g (5 oz) raspberries
100 g (3½ oz) blueberries
200 g (7 oz) cherries
1 kg (2 lb) watermelon
14–16 strawberries
12 mint leaves

Refrigerator / Freezer
2 tablespoons orange juice
100 ml (3½ fl oz) apple juice
300 ml (½ pint) pineapple juice
150 ml (¼ pint) natural yogurt
150 ml (¼ pint) lemon- or orange-
    flavoured yogurt
900 ml (1½ pints) semi-skimmed
    milk
4 tablespoons natural fromage fra
2 large scoops vanilla ice cream

Storecupboard
spirulina, wheatgrass or chlorella
clear honey or maple syrup
50 g (2 oz) muesli
organic cocoa powder
cocoa nibs

WEIGHT MANAGEMENT
JUICE RECIPES

MONDAY
minty apple tea
BENEFIT: satiating

TUESDAY
pear, grapefruit & celery juice
BENEFIT: low GI

WEDNESDAY
watermelon & raspberry juice
BENEFIT: stimulates metabolism

THURSDAY
pineapple, grape & celery juice
BENEFIT: cholesterol- & sodium-free

FRIDAY
celery & celeriac juice
BENEFIT: low carb & high fibre

SATURDAY
carrot, chilli & pineapple juice
BENEFIT: anti-inflammatory*
*Capsaicin in chilli may help reduce arthritic pain.

SUNDAY
green goddess juice
BENEFIT: reduces cholesterol*
*Lowering cholesterol brings many health
benefits, such as reducing the risk of
heart disease.

SHOPPING LIST

Fresh Fruit / Veg
5 apples, about 500 g
   (1 lb) in total
75 g (3 oz) grapefruit
275 g (9 oz) lettuce
250 g (8 oz) celery
50 g (2 oz) pear
300 g (10 oz) watermelon
125 g (4 oz) raspberries
375 g (12 oz) pineapple
125 g (4 oz) green grapes
150 g (5 oz) celeriac
100 g (3½ oz) spinach
250 g (8 oz) carrots
150 g (5 oz) broccoli
½ small chilli
½ lime
15 g (½ oz) coriander leaves
large handful of mint

Refrigerator / Freezer
200 ml (7 fl oz) chilled mint tea

Storecupboard
avocado oil

DETOX
SMOOTHIE RECIPES

MONDAY
orange & apricot super smoothie
BENEFIT: eases constipation

TUESDAY
banana & fig smoothie
BENEFIT: softens stools

WEDNESDAY
probiotic smoothie
BENEFIT: improves digestion

THURSDAY
shocking pink smoothie
BENEFIT: cleansing

FRIDAY
prune, apple & cinnamon smoothie
BENEFIT: supports gut bacteria

SATURDAY
creamy peach smoothie
BENEFIT: probiotics

SUNDAY
papaya, orange & banana smoothie
BENEFIT: supports colon cleanse

SHOPPING LIST

Fresh Fruit / Veg
1 large carrot + 250 g (8 oz)
    carrots
4 oranges
3 ripe bananas
1 fresh or dried apricot
fresh root ginger
100 g (3½ oz) figs
1 mango, about 200 g (7 oz)
1 beetroot, about 125 g (4 oz)
150 g (5 oz) blueberries
85 g (3¼ oz) strawberries
60 g (2¼ oz) raspberries
1 large peach
1 ripe papaya

Refrigerator / Freezer
200 g (7 oz) kefir
300 ml (½ pint) milk
350 ml (12 fl oz) apple juice
Greek yogurt
150 ml (¼ pint) natural yogurt
50 ml (2 fl oz) milk
300 ml (½ pint) apple juice

Storecupboard
flaked almonds
65 g (2½ oz) ready-to-eat prunes
ground cinnamon

DETOX
JUICE RECIPES

MONDAY
spicy beet juice
BENEFIT: supports waste elimination

TUESDAY
tomato, lemon & parsley juice
BENEFIT: cleansing

WEDNESDAY
spinach, celery & cucumber juice
BENEFIT: mild diuretic

THURSDAY
fabulous fennel juice
BENEFIT: relieves gas

FRIDAY
watercress & pepper punch
BENEFIT: blood cleanse

SATURDAY
broccoli, parsnip & apple juice
BENEFIT: toxin removal

SUNDAY
green lemonade
BENEFIT: enhances kidney function

SHOPPING LIST

Fresh Fruit / Veg
2 beetroot, about 300 g (10 oz)
15 g (½ oz) coriander leaves
4 celery sticks
4 tomatoes
large handful of parsley
50 g (2 oz) green pepper
50 g (2 oz) celery
55 g (2¼ oz) spinach
450 g (14½ oz) cucumber
100 g (3½ oz) tomatoes
1 fennel bulb, about 150 g (5 oz)
2 apples, about 150 g (5 oz)
1 red pepper, about 175 g (6 oz)
3 carrots, about 450 g (15 oz)
50 g (2 oz) watercress
50 g (2 oz) parsnips
150 g (5 oz) broccoli
3 lemons

Refrigerator / Freezer
sparkling water

Storecupboard
ground turmeric
grated nutmeg

ALMOND MILK & BANANA SMOOTHIE

Serves 4

½ lime
150 g (5 oz) banana
1 tablespoon peanut butter
300 ml (½ pint) almond milk
grated nutmeg, to sprinkle

Roughly peel and then juice the lime. Peel the banana.

Transfer the lime juice and banana to a food processor or blender, add the peanut butter and almond milk and process until smooth.

Pour the smoothie into 4 glasses, sprinkle with a large pinch of nutmeg and serve immediately.

For peanut butter & blueberry smoothie
Roughly peel and juice ½ lime. Transfer the juice to a food processor or blender, add 100 g (3½ oz) blueberries, 1 tablespoon peanut butter and 300 ml (½ pint) milk and process until smooth.

ALMONDS are a good source of vitamin E, an antioxidant that helps protect skin from the damaging effects of free radicals caused by pollution and other factors.

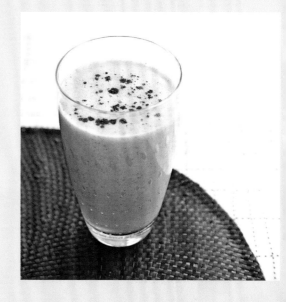

CREAMY GREEN SMOOTHIE

Serves 2

1 avocado

1 lime

30 g (1¼ oz) spinach

2 celery sticks, plus extra
  to decorate

1 garlic clove

25 g (1 oz) parsley

1 teaspoon green powder
  (such as spirulina,
  wheatgrass or chlorella)

salt and pepper

Peel and stone the avocado. Roughly peel the lime. Juice the lime with the spinach.

Transfer the avocado and the juice to a food processor or blender, add the remaining ingredients and enough water to just cover, and process until smooth. Season the smoothie to taste with salt and pepper and process again.

Pour the smoothie into 2 glasses, add a trimmed celery stick to each glass and serve immediately.

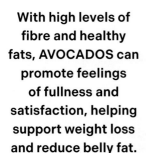

With high levels of fibre and healthy fats, AVOCADOS can promote feelings of fullness and satisfaction, helping support weight loss and reduce belly fat.

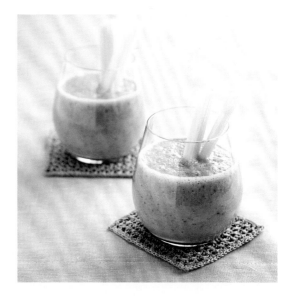

PINEAPPLE & ALFALFA JUICE

Serves 1

150 g (5 oz) pineapple

150 g (5 oz) **alfalfa sprouts,**
plus extra to decorate

2–3 ice cubes

50 ml (2 fl oz) still water

Peel and core the pineapple, chop the flesh into cubes and juice.

Transfer the pineapple juice to a food processor or blender, add the alfalfa sprouts, ice cubes and still water and process briefly.

Pour the juice into a glass, sprinkle with extra alfalfa sprouts and serve immediately.

For pineapple & lettuce juice
Juice 125 g (4 oz) pineapple with double the amount of lettuce. If you prefer a really slushy drink, blend the resulting juice with some ice cubes.

**Plant compounds
called saponins in
ALFALFA SPROUTS
have been shown
to lower LDL, or
'unhealthy' cholesterol,
decreasing the risk
of heart disease
and stroke.**

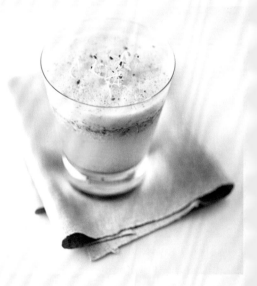

BLUEBERRY, APPLE & GINGER JUICE

Serves 1

2.5 cm (1 inch) piece fresh
   root ginger, plus extra
   to serve (optional)
250 g (8 oz) blueberries
125 g (4 oz) grapefruit
250 g (8 oz) **apples**
ice cubes (optional)

Peel and roughly chop the ginger. Juice the blueberries, grapefruit and apples with the ginger.

Pour the juice into a glass over ice, if using, decorate with thin slices of ginger, if liked, and serve immediately.

For apple & ginger juice
Juice 250 g (8 oz) apples with 2.5 cm (1 inch) ginger. If you like, top it up with ice-cold water.

APPLES are high in pectin, a fibre that turns to gel which, when combined with water in the gut, may help to ease constipation.

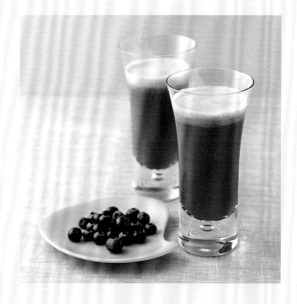

BLACKBERRY, APPLE & CELERIAC JUICE

Serves 1

100 g (3½ oz) celeriac

50 g (2 oz) apple

100 g (3½ oz) frozen **blackberries**, plus extra to decorate

2–3 ice cubes

Peel the celeriac. Juice the celeriac with the apple.

Transfer the juice to a food processor or blender, add the blackberries and the ice cubes and process briefly.

Pour the juice into a glass, decorate with extra blackberries and serve immediately.

For blackberry & pineapple juice
Juice 150 g (5 oz) each of blackberries and pineapple with 25 g (1 oz) apple. Serve in a tall glass over ice.

BLACKBERRIES are a good source of ellagic acid, an antioxidant that may help reduce damage to the skin from overexposure to the sun.

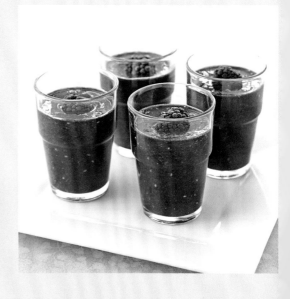

PEACH & TOFU SMOOTHIE

Serves 2

100 g (3½oz) peach
100 g (3½ oz) **tofu**
50 g (2 oz) vanilla coconut
   ice cream
100 ml (3½ fl oz) still water
few drops of natural
   almond essence
ice cubes (optional)

Halve the peach, remove the skin and stone and roughly chop the peach flesh.

Put the peach in a food processor or blender and add the tofu and ice cream. Pour in the water, add a little almond essence and process until smooth.

Pour the mixture into 2 short glasses over ice, if using, and serve immediately.

For banana & vanilla smoothie
Place 1 ripe banana, 2 teaspoons vanilla extract, 300 ml (½ pint) of plant-based (dairy-free) milk; 1 tablespoon flaxseed in a food processor or blender and blend together.

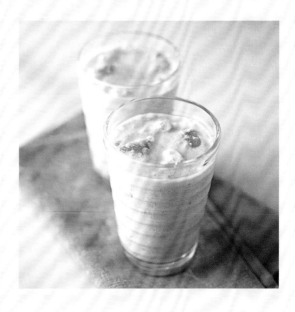

Made from soya milk, TOFU is a complete protein containing all the essential amino acids your body needs to keep muscles and bones healthy.

ORANGE & APRICOT SUPER SMOOTHIE

Serves 1

1 large **carrot**
1 orange
100 g (3½ oz) banana
+ 1 fresh or **dried apricot**
2–3 ice cubes

Juice the carrot and orange together.

Transfer the juice to a food processor or blender, add the banana, apricot and ice cubes and blend briefly.

Pour the smoothie into a glass and serve immediately.

For orange & banana smoothie
Place 1 banana, 150 ml (¼ pint) fresh orange juice and 25 g (1 oz) sunflower seeds in a food processor or blender and blend together.

APRICOTS are naturally high in fibre and sorbitol, a sugar with a laxative effect that may help promote bowel movements and relieve constipation.

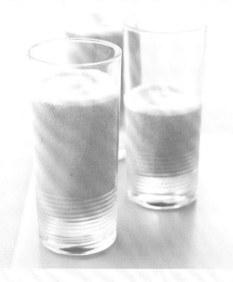

BLUEBERRY & MINT SMOOTHIE

Serves 1

100 g (3½ oz) frozen
   blueberries
150 ml (¼ pint) soya milk
small bunch of mint

Put the blueberries in a food processor or blender and pour in the soya milk. Pull the mint leaves off their stalks, reserving one or two sprigs for decoration, and add the remainder to the blender. Process briefly.

Pour the smoothie into a glass, decorate with the reserved mint sprigs and serve immediately.

For blueberry & apple smoothie
Process 250 g (8 oz) apples with 125 g (4 oz) blueberries in a food processor or blender until smooth.

Abundant in BLUEBERRIES, pterostilbene is a powerful antioxidant believed to support brain health, improving focus and memory.

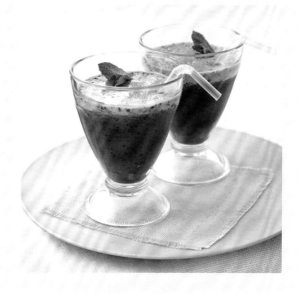

MINTY APPLE TEA

Serves 2

+ 3 **apples**, about 300 g (10 oz) in total
large handful of mint, plus extra sprigs to decorate
200 ml (7 fl oz) chilled mint tea
ice cubes

Juice the apples and mint. Stir in the chilled mint tea.

Pour the combined juice and tea into glasses over ice, decorate with a sprig of mint and serve.

For cinnamon apple tea
Juice 4 apples – about 400 g (13 oz) in total. Stir in 200 ml (7 fl oz) chilled tea, add a large pinch of ground cinnamon and stir to combine. Serve poured over crushed ice with a cinnamon stick for stirring.

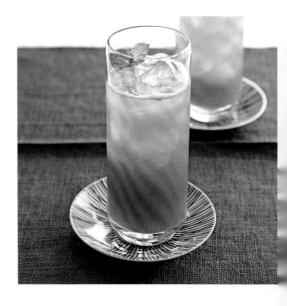

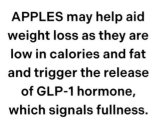

APPLES may help aid weight loss as they are low in calories and fat and trigger the release of GLP-1 hormone, which signals fullness.

BEET TREAT JUICE

Serves 1

1 slice pineapple, about
   100 g (3½ oz), plus a
   pineapple wedge
   to decorate
1 orange, about 200 g (7 oz)
2 **beetroots**, about 300 g
   (10 oz) in total
100 g (3½ oz) red cabbage

Roughly peel the pineapple and the orange. Juice all the ingredients together.

Pour the juice into a glass, decorate with a wedge of pineapple and serve immediately.

For sweet beet treat juice
Juice 2 beetroots – about 300 g (10 oz) in total, with 2 oranges – about 400 g (13 oz) in total, 1 slice roughly peeled pineapple – about 100 g (3½ oz) – and 2 peeled kiwifruits.

Nitrates, found in BEETROOT, increase blood flow and improve athletic performance by promoting oxygen delivery to the muscles.

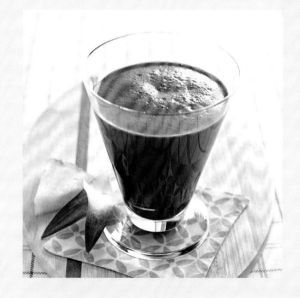

MINTY SUMMER JUICE

Serves 1

6 asparagus spears
½ cucumber, about 175 g (6 oz)
2 young carrots, about
200 g (7 oz)
small handful of mint, plus an
extra mint sprig to decorate
ice cubes

Juice together the asparagus, cucumber, carrots and mint.

Pour the juice into a glass over ice, top with a sprig of mint and serve immediately.

For spicy summer juice
Juice 6 asparagus spears with ½ cucumber – about 175 g (6 oz), 1 apple – about 100 g (3½ oz) – and a 2 cm (¾ inch) piece peeled fresh root ginger.

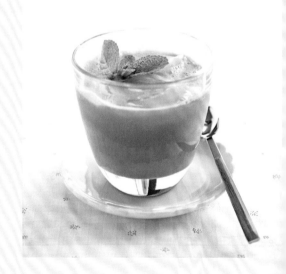

ASPARAGUS contains inulin, a prebiotic that stimulates the growth of friendly gut bacteria, promoting good digestive health.

BANANA, ORANGE & MANGO SMOOTHIE

Serves 2

1 ripe **banana**

1 ripe mango

200 ml (7 fl oz) orange juice

200 ml (7 fl oz) semi-skimmed milk

3 tablespoons fromage frais

ice cubes (optional)

Peel and slice the banana. Peel the mango, remove the stone and cut the flesh into even-sized pieces.

Put the banana and mango in a food processor or blender, add the orange juice, milk and fromage frais and process until smooth.

Pour the smoothie into 2 glasses over ice, if using, and serve immediately.

For banana & avocado smoothie
Process 1 small ripe banana with 1 small ripe avocado and 250 ml (8 fl oz) skimmed milk.

A tropical fruit, BANANAS are high in potassium, which helps to lower blood pressure and reduce the risk of heart disease.

You can swap the milk and fromage frais for any kind of plant-based alternatives, such as oat, coconut, soya, etc.

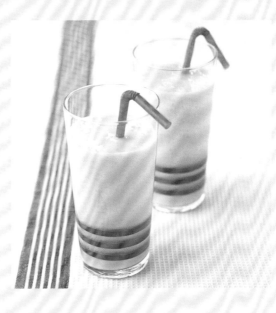

MANGO, APPLE & BLACKCURRANT SMOOTHIE

Serves 2

3 mangoes
2 tablespoons mango sorbet
100 ml (3½ fl oz) apple juice
+ 200 g (7 oz) **blackcurrants**

Peel the mangoes, remove the stones and roughly chop the flesh. Purée the mangoes with the mango sorbet and half the apple juice. Set aside to chill.

Purée the blackcurrants with the rest of the apple juice.

Spoon the mango smoothie into 2 short glasses. Place a spoon on the surface of the mango, holding it as flat as you can, and pour on the blackcurrant purée. Drag a teaspoon or skewer down the inside of the glass, to make vertical stripes around the glass.

Weight-for-weight, BLACKCURRANTS, compared to oranges, have three times the amount of vitamin C, which helps support immunity and heal wounds faster.

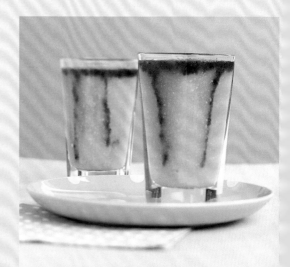

GREEN GODDESS JUICE

Serves 1

150 g (5 oz) broccoli
2 celery sticks
2 apples, about 200 g (7 oz)
10 g (⅓ oz) coriander leaves
1–2 teaspoons **avocado oil**

Juice the broccoli with the celery, apples and coriander.

Stir in the avocado oil.

Pour into a glass and serve immediately.

For green refresher juice
Juice 150 g (5 oz) broccoli with 2 celery sticks, 200 g (7 oz) peeled watermelon and ½ cucumber – about 175 g (6 oz). Serve poured over ice.

A heart-healthy food, high in monosaturated fats AVOCADO OIL may help balance blood lipids, and reduce cholesterol levels.

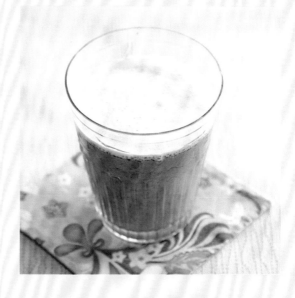

STRAWBERRY, CARROT & BEETROOT JUICE

Serves 1

- 250 g (8 oz) **carrots**
- 125 g (4 oz) beetroots
- 1 orange
- 125 g (4 oz) strawberries, plus extra to serve (optional)
- ice cubes

Juice the carrots, beetroots and orange.

Hull the strawberries. Put the carrot, beetroot and orange juice in a food processor or blender, add the strawberries and a few ice cubes and process until smooth.

Pour the juice into a large glass, decorate with a strawberry, if liked, and serve immediately.

For strawberry, melon & cucumber juice
Hull 100 g (3½ oz) strawberries and juice with 75 g (3 oz) honeydew melon and the same amount of cucumber.

Found in CARROTS, beta-carotene, a naturally occurring pigment, is converted by the body to vitamin A, which nourishes the eyes and improves night vision.

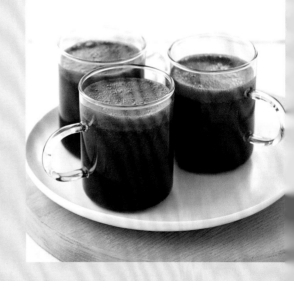

TOMATO, APPLE & BASIL JUICE

Serves 1

1 celery stick
4 large tomatoes
1 apple
ice cubes
4 **basil** leaves, finely chopped
1 ½ tablespoons lime juice
extra basil leaves, to serve
   (optional)

Trim the celery and cut it into 5 cm (2 inch) lengths. Juice the tomatoes and apple with the celery.

Pour the juice into a glass over ice, stir in the basil leaves and lime juice, shred extra basil leaves and add, if liked. Serve immediately.

For tomato, cauliflower & carrot juice
Trim 100 g (3½ oz) cauliflower and juice with 1 large tomato and 200 g (7 oz) carrots.

Essential oils found in BASIL, such as eugenol, linalool and citronellol, have shown potential therapeutic effects in treating inflammatory disorders.

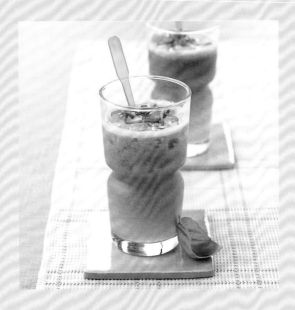

BANANA & PINEAPPLE SMOOTHIE

Serves 3

+ 1 large **banana**, plus extra to serve (optional)
  1 large ripe mango
> 150 ml (¼ pint) natural yogurt
  300 ml (½ pint) pineapple juice

Peel and slice the banana, then put it in a freezer container and freeze for at least 2 hours or overnight.

Peel the mango, remove the stone and cut the flesh into cubes.

Put the frozen banana, mango, yogurt and pineapple juice into a food processor or blender, then process until smooth.

Pour the mixture into 3 glasses, decorate with a slice of banana, if liked, and serve immediately.

The starches in BANANAS help to prevent hunger, making this popular fruit a useful food to include in a weight management programme.

You can also use a plant-based yogurt such as oat, coconut, soya, etc.

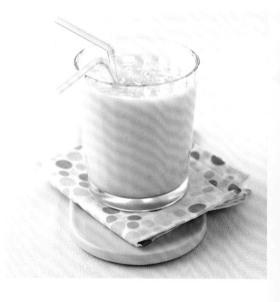

CHERRY & CHOCOLATE SMOOTHIE

Serves 2

100 g (3½ oz) blueberries
200 g (7 oz) **cherries**
1 tablespoon cocoa nibs,
    plus extra to sprinkle
300 ml (½ pint) milk

Juice the blueberries. Stone the cherries.

Transfer the blueberry juice and cherries to a food processor or blender, add the cocoa nibs and milk and process until smooth.

Pour the smoothie into 2 glasses, sprinkle with some extra cocoa nibs and serve immediately.

For breakfast cherry & chocolate smoothie
Follow the recipe above, adding 1 tablespoon cashew nuts and 1 tablespoon rolled oats to the food processor or blender with the other ingredients.

Quercetin in CHERRIES has been found to lower the levels of uric acid in the body and therefore may help to decrease the risk of developing gout.

Swap cow's milk for any kind of plant-based milk, such as oat, coconut, soya, etc.

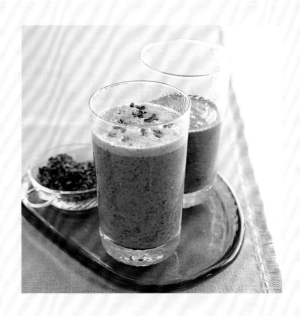

CITRUS BEET JUICE

Serves 2

1 orange, about 160 g (5½ oz)
1 beetroot, about 125 g (4 oz)
1 large carrot, about 150 g
   (5 oz), plus extra to decorate
½ cucumber, about 175 g (6 oz)

Roughly peel the orange. Juice the orange with the beetroot, carrot and cucumber.

Pour the juice into 2 glasses, decorate with slices of carrot and serve immediately.

For spicy citrus beet juice
Follow the recipe above, adding a 2 cm (¾ inch) piece peeled fresh root ginger to the juicer with the other ingredients.

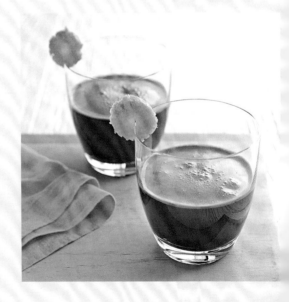

BEETROOTS contain betalains, powerful antioxidants that fight cell damage and inflammation, helping to keep the heart and arteries healthy.

BROCCOLI, PARSNIP & APPLE JUICE

Serves 1

50 g (2 oz) parsnip
50 g (2 oz) apple
150 g (5 oz) **broccoli**
2–3 ice cubes

Peel the parsnip and cut the flesh into chunks. Quarter the apple and trim the broccoli. Juice the parsnip with the apple and broccoli.

Transfer the juice to a food processor or blender and process with the ice cubes to make a creamy juice.

Pour into a glass and serve immediately.

For broccoli, carrot & beetroot juice
Trim 250 g (8 oz) broccoli and juice it with 175 g (6 oz) carrots and 50 g (2 oz) beetroot.

By supporting the liver in removing harmful toxins, sulphoraphane, a chemical found in BROCCOLI, has been found to reduce the action of cancer-causing agents.

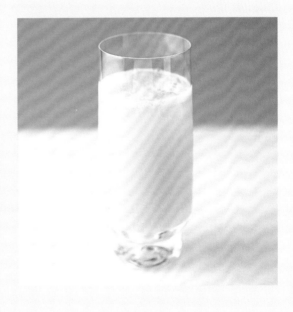

COOL CURRANTS JUICE

Serves 1

2 apples, about 200 g (7 oz)
   in total
 300 g (10 oz) blackcurrants
100 g (3½ oz) redcurrants
sprig of blackcurrants or
   redcurrants, to decorate

Juice all the ingredients together.

Pour the juice into a glass, decorate with
a sprig of currants and serve immediately.

For currant & berry juice
Replace 100 g (3½ oz) of the blackcurrants
with 100 g (3½ oz) mixed strawberries and
blackberries and juice as above.

BLACKCURRANTS
have a high anthocyanin
content, a natural
pigment associated
with improved vision,
and a decreased feeling
of tired eyes.

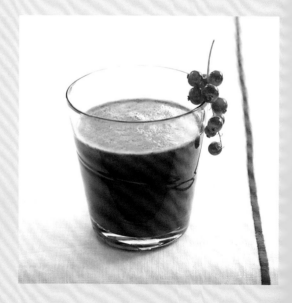

SHOCKING PINK SMOOTHIE

Serves 2

1 **beetroot**, about 125 g (4 oz)
1 banana
85 g (3¼ oz) strawberries,
    plus extra to decorate
60 g (2¼ oz) raspberries
1 tablespoon flaked almonds
300 ml (½ pint) milk
ice cubes

Juice the beetroot. Peel the banana.

Transfer the beetroot juice and banana to a food processor or blender, add the berries, almonds and milk and process until smooth.

Pour the smoothie into 2 tall glasses over ice, decorate with strawberries and serve immediately.

For shocking pink protein boost
Follow the recipe above, adding 2 tablespoons whey protein powder to the food processor or blender with the other ingredients. If the smoothie is a little too thick, just add another dash of milk.

BEETROOTS contain glutathione, a detoxifying antioxidant that helps the liver neutralize and excrete toxins.

You can also use a plant-based milk such as oat, coconut, soya, etc.

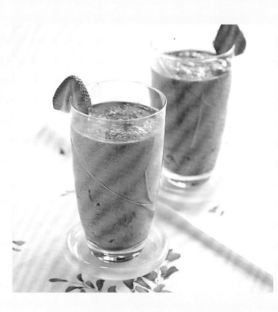

CUCUMBER, LEMON & MINT SMOOTHIE

Serves 1

+ 250 g (8 oz) **cucumber**,
    plus extra to serve
  ½ **lemon**
  3–4 fresh mint leaves
  2–3 ice cubes

Peel and roughly chop the cucumber. Squeeze the lemon.

Put the cucumber and lemon into a food processor or blender with the mint leaves and ice cubes and process briefly.

Pour into a tall glass, decorate with a strip of cucumber, if liked, and serve immediately.

For grapefruit & cucumber crush
Chop 1 cucumber and blend it with 150 ml (¼ pint) grapefruit juice and a handful of ice cubes. Process the ingredients to make an ice-cold slushy drink.

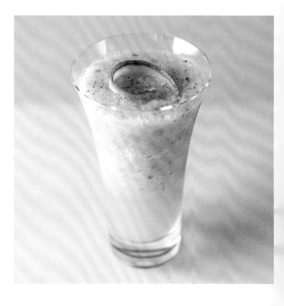

CUCUMBERS are water-rich, so they can help improve hydration and keep our concentration and energy levels up.

FOREST FRUITS JUICE

Serves 1

200 g (7 oz) **blackberries**
100 g (3½ oz) blueberries
1 apple, about 100 g (3½ oz)

Juice all the ingredients together.

Pour into a glass and serve immediately.

For green forest fruits juice
Juice 1 apple – about 100 g (3½ oz) – with
200 g (7 oz) blackberries, 30 g (1¼ oz) kale and
a 2 cm (¾ inch) piece peeled fresh root ginger.

**Found in
BLACKBERRIES,
salicylic acid has
properties similar to
aspirin, which could help
lower blood pressure
and protect against
heart disease.**

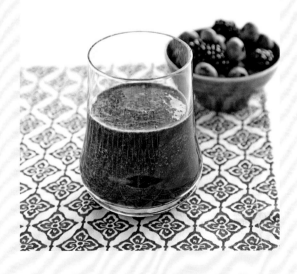

FENNEL & CAMOMILE JUICE

Serves 1

1 lemon, plus extra to decorate

150 g (5 oz) fennel bulb

100 ml (3½ fl oz) chilled
   camomile tea

ice cubes

Roughly peel the lemon and juice it with the fennel. Mix the juice with the chilled camomile tea.

Pour the combined juice and tea into a glass over ice and serve with slices of lemon, to decorate.

For fennel & lettuce juice
Juice 125 g (4 oz) fennel bulb and 175 g (6 oz) lettuce with ½ lemon. Pour into a glass over ice and decorate with a slice of lemon.

**CAMOMILE TEA
contains active
compounds, including
apigenin, that help calm
the nervous system
and relieve tension
and irritability.**

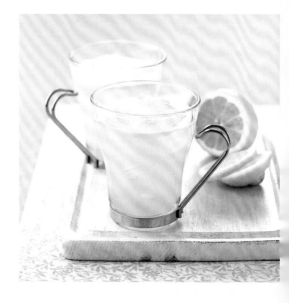

BROCCOLI, SPINACH & APPLE JUICE

Serves 1

150 g (5 oz) **broccoli**

150 g (5 oz) spinach

2 apples

2–3 ice cubes

Trim the broccoli and rinse the spinach. Juice the apples with the spinach and broccoli, alternating the spinach leaves with the other ingredients so that the spinach leaves do not clog the machine.

Transfer the juice to a food processor or blender, add a couple of ice cubes and process briefly.

Pour into a glass and serve immediately.

For spinach, apple & pepper juice
Increase the apple to 250 g (8 oz) and, instead of broccoli, juice 100 g (3½ oz) yellow pepper. Stir in a pinch of ground cinnamon to serve.

BROCCOLI is a good source of calcium, which is important for healthy bone development and preventing bone disorders.

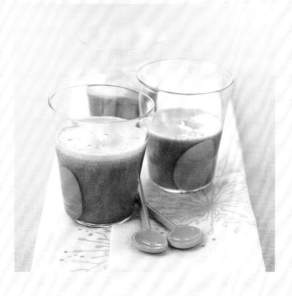

MANDARIN & LYCHEE FRAPPÉ

Serves 1

100 g (3½ oz) mandarin
  oranges, canned in
  natural juice
 50 g (2 oz) lychees, canned
  in natural juice
ice cubes

Put the oranges and lychees and the juices
from the cans into a food processor or
blender, add the ice cubes and process briefly.

Pour into a glass and serve immediately.

For ruby smoothie

Put the juice of 2 oranges and 1 apple in a food
processor or blender with 150 g (5 oz) each
raspberries and strawberries. Add 150 ml
(¼ pint) natural yogurt and process briefly.

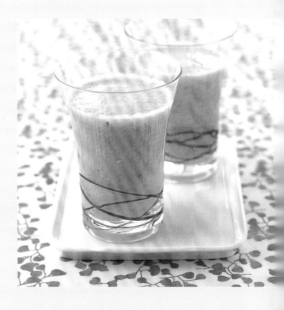

**A sweet and hydrating
fruit, LYCHEES provide
a natural energy boost
and a refreshing
floral flavour.**

KIWIFRUIT, MANGO & RASPBERRY SMOOTHIE

Serves 2

3 kiwifruits

150 ml (¼ pint) lemon- or
  orange-flavoured yogurt

1 small **mango**, peeled, stoned
  and roughly chopped

2 tablespoons orange juice

150 g (5 oz) raspberries

1–2 teaspoons clear honey
  (optional)

**Low in fat and high in fibre,
MANGOES may help curb
hunger, regulate blood
sugar levels and aid with
weight loss.**

V

**You can also use a plant-
based yogurt such as
oat, coconut, soya, etc.
Swap honey for maple or
agave syrup if vegan.**

Peel and roughly chop the kiwifruit, then process in a food processor or blender until smooth. Spoon the purée into 2 tall glasses, and top each with a spoonful of yogurt, spreading the yogurt to the sides of the glasses.

Blend the mango to a purée with the orange juice and spoon it into the glasses on top of the kiwifruit purée and yogurt. Top with another layer of yogurt.

Blend the raspberries and push them through a sieve over a bowl to extract the seeds. Check their sweetness (you might need to stir in a little honey if they're very sharp) and spoon the raspberry purée into the glasses.

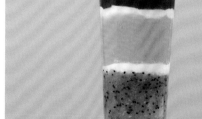

CARROT & BRUSSELS JUICE

Serves 1

2 cm (¾ inch) piece fresh
   root ginger

 6 Brussels sprouts

1 carrot, about 150 g (5 oz)

1 apple, about 100 g (3½ oz)

Peel the ginger. Juice all the ingredients together.

Pour into a glass and serve immediately.

For celery & Brussels juice
Juice 10 Brussels sprouts with 2 celery sticks, 1 carrot – about 150 g (5 oz), 100 g (3½ oz) broccoli and 1 apple – about 100 g (3½ oz).

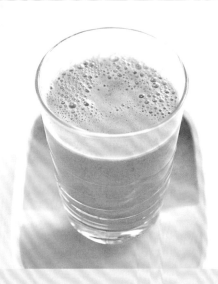

BRUSSELS SPROUTS are rich in a plant compound called kaempferol, an antioxidant that may be used to treat inflammation-induced conditions.

SPINACH, CELERY & CUCUMBER JUICE

Serves 1

50 g (2 oz) green pepper

50 g (2 oz) **celery**

25 g (1 oz) spinach

100 g (3½ oz) cucumber

100 g (3½ oz) tomatoes, plus
   extra to serve (optional)

salt and pepper

ice cubes (optional)

Core and deseed the pepper. Trim the celery and cut it into 5 cm (2 inch) lengths. Juice the spinach, cucumber and tomatoes with the pepper and celery. Season the juice to taste with salt and pepper.

Pour the juice into a glass over ice, if using, decorate with tomato quarters, if liked, and serve immediately.

For kale & spirulina juice
Juice 25 g (1 oz) kale with 100 g (3½ oz) wheatgrass. Stir in 1 teaspoon spirulina before serving. This unusual-tasting juice offers excellent health benefits.

**CELERY is mildly diuretic
due to butylphthalide,
which increases urine
production, helping to
remove excess water
and salt.**

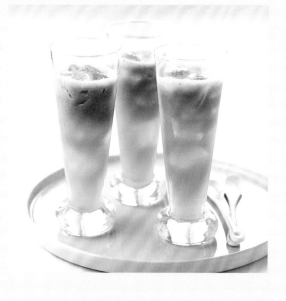

CARROT, FENNEL & GINGER JUICE

Serves 1

2.5 cm (1 inch) piece fresh
   root ginger

75 g (3 oz) celery

 300 g (10 oz) **carrots**

50 g (2 oz) fennel, plus extra
   to serve (optional)

1 tablespoon spirulina
   (optional)

ice cubes (optional)

fennel fronds, to decorate
   (optional)

Peel and roughly chop the ginger. Trim the celery and cut it into 5 cm (2 inch) lengths. Juice the carrots, fennel and spirulina, if using, with the ginger and celery.

Pour the juice into a glass over ice, if using, decorate with strips of fennel and fennel fronds, if liked, and serve immediately.

For carrot, apple & ginger juice
Peel and roughly chop 1 cm (½ inch) cube fresh root ginger and juice it with 2 carrots and 1 tart apple, such as a Granny Smith.

CARROTS are a rich vegetable source of beta-carotene known to help protect against high blood cholesterol and heart disease.

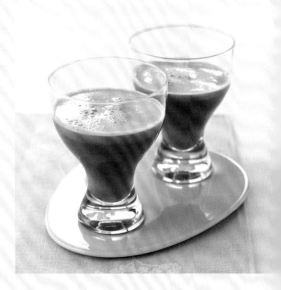

RED PEPPER & TOMATO SMOOTHIE

Serves 1

50 g (2 oz) **red pepper**
50 g (2 oz) cucumber
30 g (1¼ oz) spring onion
100 ml (3½ fl oz) tomato juice
splash of lemon juice
splash of hot pepper sauce
splash of Worcestershire
    sauce
salt and pepper

Core and deseed the red pepper and roughly chop the flesh. Peel the cucumber and roughly chop. Roughly chop the spring onion, reserving a few shreds for a garnish.

Pour the tomato juice into a food processor or blender, add the pepper, cucumber and spring onion and process briefly. Taste, then season to taste with lemon juice, hot pepper sauce, Worcestershire sauce and salt and pepper.

Pour the smoothie into a glass, garnish with the remaining spring onion and serve immediately.

RED PEPPERS are a great source of vitamin C, which can help absorb iron. Iron is often depleted in women and girls of reproductive age.

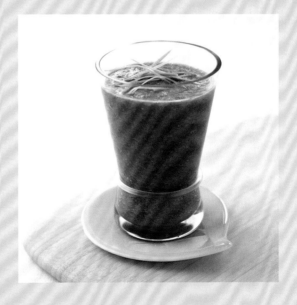

MANGO & MINT SHERBET

Serves 6

3 ripe mangoes
4 tablespoons lemon juice
 12 **mint leaves**, finely chopped
900 ml (1½ pints) ice-cold
   water
ice cubes

Peel and stone the mangoes and roughly chop the flesh.

Put it into a food processor or blender with the lemon juice, mint leaves and water and process until smooth.

Pour the smoothie into tall glasses over ice and serve immediately.

For mango & blackcurrant smoothie
Process the flesh of 3 mangoes with 100 ml (3½ fl oz) apple juice and 200 g (7 oz) blackcurrants.

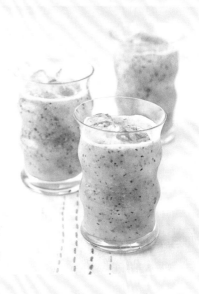

Menthol, a chemical naturally found in MINT, has an anti-spasmodic effect, calming the gut and relieving digestive discomfort.

GINGER, PEAR & CINNAMON JUICE

Serves 1

2 cm (¾ inch) piece fresh
   root ginger
5 pears, about 750 g (1½ lb)
   in total
large pinch of ground **cinnamon**
ice cubes

Peel the ginger. Juice the ginger with the pears. Stir in the cinnamon.

Pour the juice into a glass over ice and serve immediately.

For gingered mango juice
Peel a 2 cm (¾ inch) piece fresh root ginger. Peel and stone 2 mangoes – about 400 g (13 oz) in total. Juice the ginger and mangoes with 2 apples – about 200 g (7 oz) in total. Serve poured over ice.

The active ingredient in CINNAMON, cinnamaldehyde, has an insulin-like effect, lowering blood sugar levels and helping to maintain heart health.

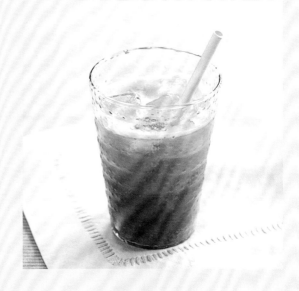

CELERY & CELERIAC JUICE

Serves 1

100 g (3½ oz) celery
150 g (5 oz) **celeriac**
100 g (3½ oz) lettuce
100 g (3½ oz) spinach
2–3 ice cubes

Trim the celery and cut it into 5 cm (2 inch) lengths. Peel the celeriac and cut the flesh into cubes. Separate the lettuce into leaves. Juice the celery, celeriac, lettuce and spinach, alternating the ingredients so that the lettuce and spinach leaves do not clog the machine.

Transfer the juice to a food processor or blender, add a couple of ice cubes and process briefly.

Pour into a tall glass and serve immediately.

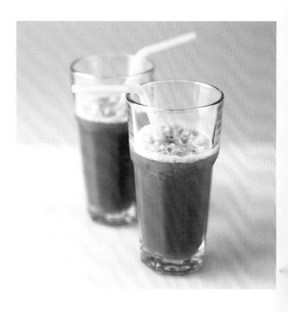

Low in carbohydrates yet high in fibre, CELERIAC may help with weight loss by decreasing appetite and cravings.

MELON, CARROT & GINGER JUICE

Serves 1

250 g (8 oz) cantaloupe melon

1 lime

1 cm (½ inch) piece fresh
   root ginger

125 g (4 oz) **carrot**

ice cubes, to serve (optional)

Peel and deseed the melon and cut the flesh into cubes. Peel the lime. Peel and roughly chop the ginger. Juice the carrot with the melon, lime and ginger.

Pour the juice into a glass over ice, if using, and serve immediately.

For carrot, orange & apple juice
Juice 2 carrots with 1 orange and 1 apple.

Beta-carotene, found in CARROTS, is beneficial for the skin. It protects against sun damage and helps prevent oxidative stress, a cause of skin ageing.

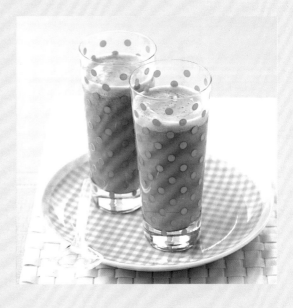

BREAKFAST NUT SMOOTHIE

Serves 2

2 oranges, about 400 g (13 oz)

1 banana

1 tablespoon muesli

 1 tablespoon **cashew nuts**

300 ml (½ pint) milk

ground cinnamon, to sprinkle

Roughly peel and juice the oranges. Peel the banana.

Transfer the orange juice and banana to a food processor or blender, add the muesli and milk and process until smooth.

Pour the smoothie into 2 glasses, sprinkle with ground cinnamon and serve immediately.

For a personalized nut breakfast smoothie
Follow the recipe above, replacing the 1 tablespoon muesli with 1 tablespoon nuts of your choice (walnuts and pecans both work really well).

CASHEW NUTS are rich in copper, a mineral that helps in the formation of red blood cells, which carry oxygen to produce energy.

Swap cow's milk for any kind of plant-based milk, such as oat, coconut, soya, etc.

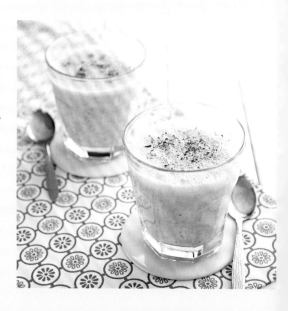

BANANA & CHOCOLATE SMOOTHIE

Serves 2

1 banana

2 tablespoons organic
  cocoa powder

300 ml (½ pint) semi-skimmed
  milk

100 ml (3½ fl oz) apple juice

2 large scoops vanilla ice cream

organic cocoa powder,
  to decorate

Peel and roughly chop the banana. Place in a food processor or blender with the cocoa powder, milk, apple juice and ice cream and process until smooth.

Pour the mixture into 2 tall glasses, dust with cocoa powder and serve.

For banana & peanut butter smoothie
Put a banana, 300 ml (½ pint) semi-skimmed milk and 1 tablespoon smooth peanut butter into a food processor or blender and process until smooth.

DARK COCOA is one of the highest plant sources of magnesium, a mineral that may help manage the body's stress response.

V

Swap the dairy milk and ice cream for any plant-based alternatives, such as oat, coconut, soya, etc.

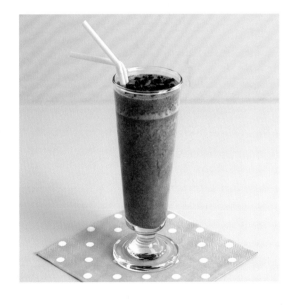

TOMATO, RED PEPPER & CABBAGE JUICE

Serves 1

175 g (6 oz) red pepper

175 g (6 oz) tomatoes

+ 100 g (3 ½ oz) **white cabbage**

1 tablespoon chopped parsley

lime wedge, to decorate
 (optional)

Core and deseed the pepper. Juice the tomatoes and cabbage with the pepper.

Pour the juice into a tall glass, stir in the parsley, decorate with a lime wedge, if liked, and serve immediately.

For tomato, red pepper & celery juice
Trim 4 celery sticks and cut them into 5 cm (2 inch) lengths. Juice the celery with 3 ripe tomatoes and half a red pepper. Add a crushed garlic clove and chopped chilli, to taste.

CABBAGE juice is a traditional remedy for stomach ulcers. It contains vitamin U, which is believed to stimulate the formation of protective gastric mucous and stomach healing.

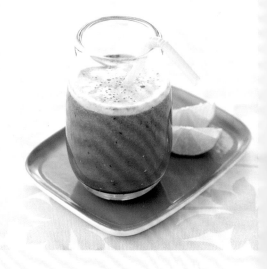

PEAR, CELERY & GINGER JUICE

Serves 1

50 g (2 oz) **celery**
2.5 cm (1 inch) piece fresh
  root ginger
100 g (3½ oz) pear
ice cubes

Trim the celery and cut it into 5 cm (2 inch) lengths. Peel and roughly chop the ginger. Juice the pear with the celery and ginger.

Pour the juice into a glass over ice. Or you can briefly process the juice in a food processor or blender with 2–3 ice cubes.

For pear & peach juice
Juice 3 pears with 2 peaches to give a thick, nutritious drink.

CELERY contains a phytochemical called phthalides, shown to relax the tissues of the artery walls, increasing blood flow and reducing blood pressure.

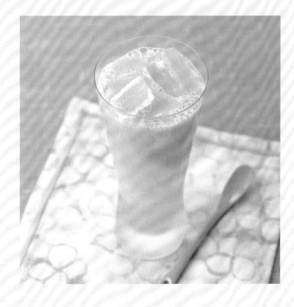

CARROT, CHILLI & PINEAPPLE JUICE

Serves 1

½ small **chilli**
250 g (8 oz) pineapple
250 g (8 oz) carrots
ice cubes
juice of ½ lime
1 tablespoon chopped
   coriander leaves

Deseed the chilli. Remove the core and peel from the pineapple. Juice the carrots with the chilli and pineapple.

Pour the juice into a glass over ice. Squeeze over the lime juice, stir in the chopped coriander and serve immediately.

For tomato, celery & ginger juice
Trim 100 g (3½ oz) celery and roughly chop 2.5 cm (1 inch) piece each of fresh root ginger and fresh horseradish. Juice the celery, ginger and horseradish with 300 g (10 oz) tomatoes, 175 g (6 oz) carrots and a garlic clove. Serve over ice, decorated with celery slivers, if liked.

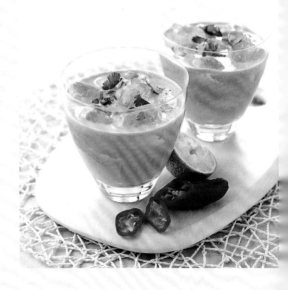

Famous for their fiery kick, CHILLIES contain capsaicin, which has pain-relieving properties and may help reduce pain and discomfort in arthritic joints.

MANGO, COCONUT & LIME LASSI

Serves 3

1 large ripe mango

juice of 1 orange, plus slices, to decorate (optional)

juice of 1 lime

1 tablespoon clear honey

300 ml (½ pint) natural yogurt

4 tablespoons **coconut milk**

ice cubes (optional)

Peel the mango, remove the stone and dice the flesh. Put the mango in a food processor or blender with the orange and lime juices, honey, yogurt and coconut milk. Process until smooth.

Transfer the mixture to a jug then pour into tall glasses over ice, if using, decorate with slices of orange, if liked, and serve immediately.

For pineapple & coconut smoothie
Process 100 g (3 ½ oz) pineapple flesh with 100 ml (3 ½ fl oz) coconut milk and 100 ml (3½ fl oz) soya milk. Serve sprinkled with toasted coconut.

COCONUT MILK contains lauric acid that can help protect the body from infections and viruses.

Swap the dairy yogurt for any kind of plant-based alternative and honey with maple or agave syrup.

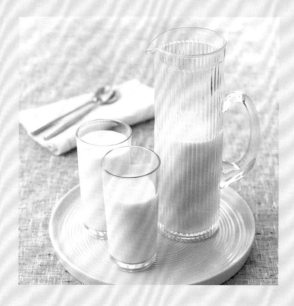

MELON, MINT & BERRY SMOOTHIE

Serves 4

+ 1 kg (2 lb) **watermelon**
14–16 strawberries
12 mint leaves
small handful of ice cubes

Peel the melon as close to the skin as possible. Hull the strawberries.

Place all the ingredients in a food processor or blender and process until smooth.

Pour into 4 glasses and serve immediately.

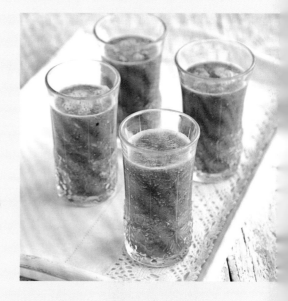

Useful for staying hydrated, WATERMELONS contain 90% water, which is highly mineralized, making them ideal for summer or post-workout.

CRANBERRY & APPLE SMOOTHIE

Serves 1

250 g (8 oz) apples
100 g (3½ oz) frozen **cranberries**
100 ml (3½ fl oz) natural yogurt
1 tablespoon clear honey
ice cubes (optional)

Juice the apples.

Transfer the juice to a food processor or blender, add the cranberries, yogurt and honey and process briefly.

Pour the smoothie into a glass over ice, if using, and serve immediately.

For grapeberry smoothie
Blend together 125 g (4 oz) blackberries, 300 ml (½ pint) purple grape juice and 3 tablespoons natural yogurt.

CRANBERRIES contain proanthocyanidins, chemical substances believed to block E.coli, the bug that commonly causes urinary tract infections.

Swap the dairy yogurt for any kind of plant-based alternative and honey with maple or agave syrup.

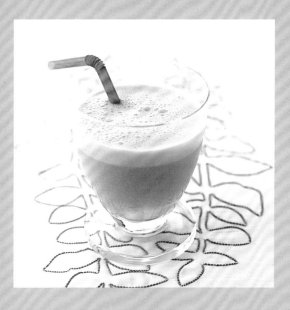

FABULOUS FENNEL JUICE

Serves 1

1 **fennel** bulb, about 150 g (5 oz)

1 apple, about 100 g (3½ oz)

1 carrot, about 150 g (5 oz)

grated nutmeg, to sprinkle

Juice all the ingredients together.

Pour the juice into a glass, sprinkle with a large pinch of nutmeg and serve immediately.

For fennel & orange juice
Roughly peel 1 orange – about 160 g (5½ oz). Juice the orange with 1 fennel bulb – about 150 g (5 oz) – and 1 carrot – about 150 g (5 oz). To add extra fibre to the juice, if desired, stir in ½ teaspoon ground flaxseeds.

The aniseed flavour of FENNEL comes from anethole, which is believed to aid digestion and relieve gas.

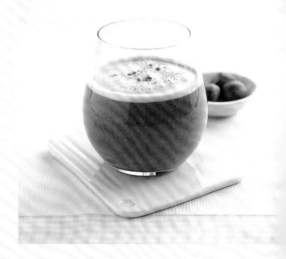

THE DAILY BOOST

SPICY BEET JUICE

Serves 1

1 large beetroot, about 175 g
   (6 oz)
15 g (½ oz) **coriander** leaves
2 celery sticks
large pinch of ground turmeric
pepper

Juice the beetroot with the coriander and celery.

Whisk in the ground turmeric. Season the juice to taste with pepper.

Pour the juice into a glass and serve immediately.

For spicy roots juice
Juice 1 parsnip – about 100 g (3½ oz), 1 carrot – about 150 g (5 oz), 1 apple – about 100 g (3½ oz) – and a 2 cm (¾ inch) piece peeled fresh root ginger. Whisk in a large pinch of ground turmeric and serve.

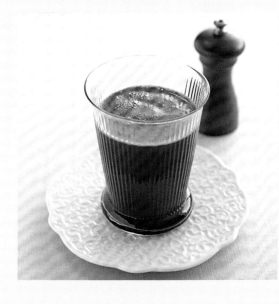

CORIANDER contains flavonoids, active compounds that bind to heavy metals, making them easier to excrete through the body.

VIRGIN PIÑA COLADA JUICE

Serves 2

400 g (13 oz) pineapple, plus
    a small pineapple wedge
    to decorate

+ 200 ml (7 fl oz) **coconut water**

ice cubes

Peel and juice the pineapple. Stir the coconut water into the pineapple juice.

Pour the combined juice and coconut water into 2 glasses over ice, decorate with a wedge of pineapple and serve immediately.

For mango & coconut juice
Juice 3 peeled and stoned mangoes – about 600 g (1 lb 3½ oz) in total. Stir in 200 ml (7 fl oz) coconut water and serve poured over ice with a slice of mango to decorate.

**High in electrolyte
minerals and glucose,
COCONUT WATER
can help hydrate,
improving the capacity
to exercise.**

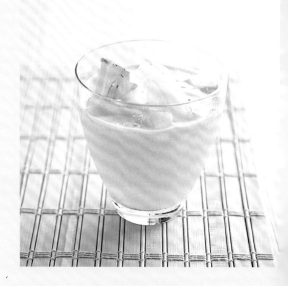

BANANA & FIG SMOOTHIE

Serves 1

2.5 cm (1 inch) piece fresh
   root ginger
100 g (3½ oz) **fig**, plus extra
   to serve (optional)
1 orange
250 g (8 oz) carrots
100 g (3½ oz) banana
ice cubes

Peel and roughly chop the ginger. Juice the fig and orange with the carrots and ginger.

Transfer the juice to a food processor or blender, add the banana and some ice cubes and process until smooth.

Pour the drink into a glass, add more ice cubes, decorate with sliced figs, if liked, and serve immediately.

For banana & papaya smoothie
Put the flesh of a papaya in a food processor or blender with a banana, the juice of 1 orange, 300 ml (½ pint) apple juice and some ice. Process until smooth.

Due to their high soluble fibre content, FIGS can promote digestive health by softening stools and decreasing constipation.

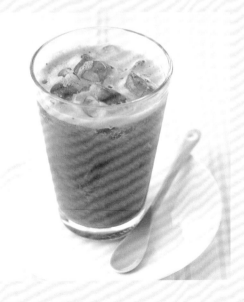

HEAVENLY HEMP SMOOTHIE

Serves 2

1 papaya, about 250 g (8 oz)

1 apricot, about 75 g (3 oz)

1 lime, plus extra to decorate

 400 ml (14 fl oz) **hemp milk**

1 teaspoon chia oil

¼ teaspoon ground cinnamon

Peel and deseed the papaya. Stone the apricot. Roughly peel and then juice the lime.

Transfer the papaya, apricot and lime juice to a food processor or blender, add the remaining ingredients and process until smooth.

Pour the smoothie into 2 glasses, add a wedge of lime to each glass and serve immediately.

For minty digestive delight smoothie
Follow the recipe above, adding 10–12 mint leaves to the food processor or blender with the other ingredients.

HEMP MILK is a good source of omega-3 and omega-6 fatty acids, which can help to reduce inflammation and improve skin health.

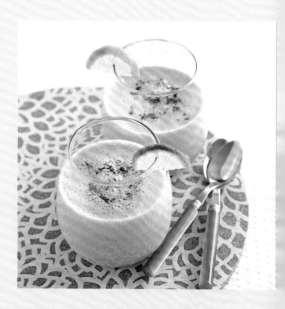

CARROT, CHICORY & CELERY JUICE

Serves 1

175 g (6 oz) carrots

125 g (4 oz) celery

125 g (4 oz) **chicory**

2–3 ice cubes

lemon slices, to serve

chopped parsley, to serve
  (optional)

Scrub the carrots. Trim the celery and cut it into 5 cm (2 inch) lengths. Juice the chicory with the carrots and celery.

Transfer the juice to a food processor or blender, add a couple of ice cubes and process briefly.

Pour the juice into a glass, decorate with slices of lemon and some chopped parsley, if liked, and serve immediately.

For carrot & cabbage juice
Juice 250 g (8 oz) each of carrots and cabbage and serve over ice. This quick juice soothes upset stomachs.

The substance lactucopicrin, which contributes to CHICORY'S bitter taste is believed to have sedative effect on the central nervous system.

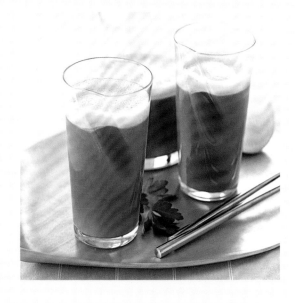

KICKSTART JUICE

Serves 1

1 lemon
2 cm (¾ inch) piece fresh
    root ginger
✚ 1 **garlic** clove
1 apple, about 100 g (3½ oz)
1 carrot, about 150 g (5 oz)
2 celery sticks
100 g (3½ oz) alfalfa sprouts

Roughly peel the lemon, ginger and garlic. Juice all the ingredients together.

Pour into a glass and serve immediately.

For clean start juice
Juice 1 roughly peeled lemon with 1 roughly peeled lime, ½ cucumber – about 175 g (6 oz) – and a 2 cm (¾ inch) piece peeled fresh root ginger. Pour the juice into a tall glass and top up with sparkling water.

The pungent odour of GARLIC comes from allicin, a compound that may help relax blood vessels, improve blood flow, and lower blood pressure.

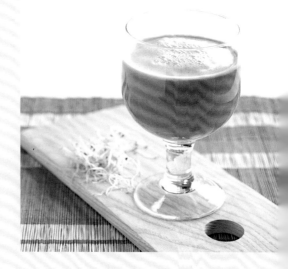

PINEAPPLE, GRAPE & CELERY JUICE

Serves 1

125 g (4 oz) pineapple

125 g (4 oz) green **grapes**

50 g (2 oz) celery

50 g (2 oz) lettuce

2–3 ice cubes (optional)

Remove the skin and core from the pineapple. Juice the pineapple with the grapes, celery and lettuce.

Pour the juice into a glass over ice, if using, and serve immediately.

For pineapple & pear juice
Double the amount of pineapple and replace the grapes, celery and lettuce with 2 pears – about 350 g (11½ oz) in total – and ½ lime.

Fat-free, cholesterol-free, and sodium-free, GRAPES are a healthy sweet treat that are helpful for weight loss.

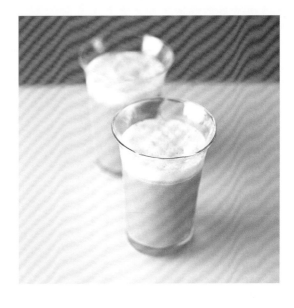

PROBIOTIC SMOOTHIE

Serves 1

1 orange, about 200 g (7 oz)
1 mango, about 200 g (7 oz)
+ 200 g (7 oz) **kefir**
150 g (5 oz) blueberries

Roughly peel and then juice the orange. Peel and stone the mango.

Transfer the orange juice and mango to a food processor or blender, add the kefir and blueberries and process until smooth.

Pour the smoothie into a glass and serve immediately.

For kefir & berry smoothie
Juice 1 roughly peeled orange – about 200 g (7 oz). Transfer the juice to a food processor or blender, add 200 g (7 oz) kefir and 150 g (5 oz) frozen mixed berries and process until smooth.

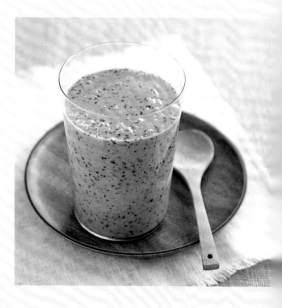

Probiotics in KEFIR could help regulate harmful bacteria, improve digestion, and even manufacture some vitamins in the gut.

RASPBERRY, KIWIFRUIT & GRAPEFRUIT SMOOTHIE

Serves 1

150 g (5 oz) grapefruit

175 g (6 oz) pineapple

50 g (2 oz) **kiwifruit**

50 g (2 oz) frozen raspberries,
plus extra to serve (optional)

50 g (2 oz) frozen cranberries

Peel and segment the grapefruit. Remove the skin and core from the pineapple. Juice the kiwifruit with the grapefruit and pineapple.

Transfer the juice to a food processor or blender, add the frozen berries and process until smooth.

Pour the smoothie into a glass, decorate with raspberries, if liked, and serve with a straw.

For strawberry & pineapple smoothie
Process 150 g (5 oz) frozen strawberries with 150 ml (¼ pint) pineapple juice and 150 ml (¼ pint) strawberry yogurt.

The distinctive green flesh of the KIWIFRUIT is packed with vitamin C, essential for producing collagen that helps keep skin smooth and firm.

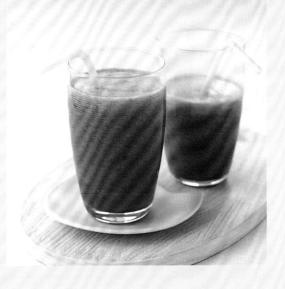

GRAPEFRUIT & ORANGE JUICE

Serves 1

½ **grapefruit**
1 large orange
1 lime
ice cubes or sparkling
  mineral water

Peel all the fruit, leaving a little of the pith on the segments. If you like, reserve some of the lime rind to decorate.

Juice the fruit, then either serve it over ice or, if you want a longer drink, dilute it with an equal amount of sparkling mineral water. Serve the juice decorated with curls of lime rind, if liked.

For orange & carrot juice
Peel and segment 2 oranges and juice with 125 g (4 oz) carrots.

The plant chemical naringenin found in GRAPEFRUITS may help lower LDL, or 'unhealthy' cholesterol, reducing the risk of heart disease and stroke.

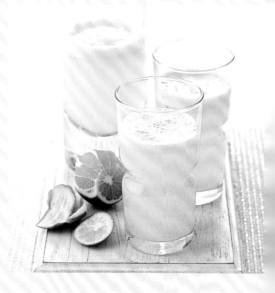

PEAR, GRAPEFRUIT & CELERY JUICE

Serves 1

75 g (3 oz) **grapefruit**
125 g (4 oz) lettuce
75 g (3 oz) celery
50 g (2 oz) pear
ice cubes (optional)

Peel the grapefruit and divide it into segments. Separate the lettuce into leaves. Trim the celery and cut it into 5 cm (2 inch) lengths. Quarter the pear. Juice the grapefruit with the lettuce, celery and pear.

Pour the juice into a glass over ice, if using, and serve immediately.

For grapefruit & lemon juice
Peel and segment a grapefruit and juice it with 5 cm (2 inches) cucumber and ½ lemon. Top up with sparkling mineral water.

GRAPEFRUITS are ideal additions to a weight management plan due to their low glycaemic index rating and high soluble fibre content, which promotes a feeling of fullness.

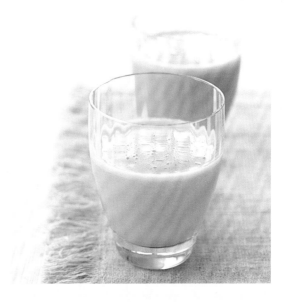

SWEET PEPPER JUICE

Serves 1

1 teaspoon ground mixed
  peppercorns
lime wedge
1 red pepper, about 175 g (6 oz)
20 red grapes
2–3 ice cubes

Place the ground peppercorns on a small plate. Rub the rim of a glass with the lime wedge and dip the rim of the glass into the peppercorns to coat the rim.

Core and deseed the red pepper. Juice the pepper with the grapes.

Transfer the juice to a food processor or blender, add the ice cubes and process briefly until smooth.

Pour the juice into the prepared glass and serve immediately.

**Piperine is an
active ingredient in
PEPPERCORNS and
is thought to increase
the absorption of
several nutrients
and beneficial
phytochemicals.**

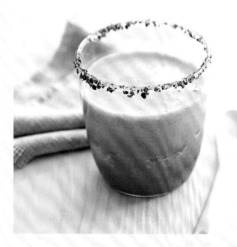

THE DAILY BOOST

MANGO, PINEAPPLE & LIME SMOOTHIE

Serves 2

1 ripe mango
300 ml (½ pint) pineapple juice
rind and juice of ½ **lime**
lime wedges, to serve
  (optional)

Peel the mango, remove the stone, roughly chop the flesh and put it in a freezer container. Freeze for at least 2 hours or overnight.

Put the frozen mango in a food processor or blender, add the pineapple juice and lime rind and juice and process until thick.

Pour the smoothie into 2 short glasses, decorate with lime wedges, if liked, and serve immediately.

For apricot & pineapple smoothie
Soak 65 g (2½ oz) dried apricots overnight in 350 ml (12 fl oz) pineapple juice. Process the mixture with some ice until smooth.

Hesperidin, a flavonoid found in LIMES, has been shown to have therapeutic potential in heart disease, reducing symptoms of high blood pressure.

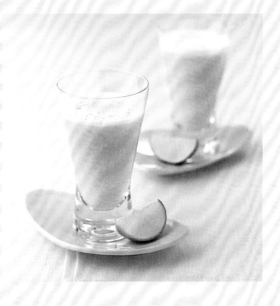

NECTARINE & RASPBERRY YOGURT SMOOTHIE

Serves 2

✚ 3 **nectarines**, about 450 g
   (14½ oz)
   175 g (6 oz) raspberries
❯ 150 ml (¼ pint) natural yogurt
   handful of ice cubes

Halve and stone the nectarines.

Put the nectarines and raspberries in a food processor or blender and process until really smooth. Add the yogurt and process again, then add the ice and process until very crushed and the shake thickens.

Pour into 2 chilled glasses. Decorate with cocktail umbrellas and anything else to make the drink look fun!

NECTARINES are a good source of the antioxidant lutein, which helps fight free radical damage and supports healthy skin, improving hydration and elasticity.

You can also use a plant-based yogurt such as oat, coconut, soya, etc.

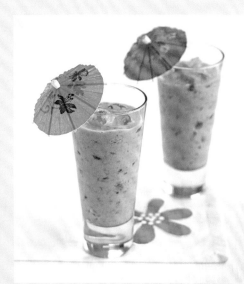

TOMATO, CARROT & GINGER JUICE

Serves 1

2.5 cm (1 inch) cube fresh
   root **ginger**

100 g (3½ oz) celery, plus extra
   to serve (optional)

300 g (10 oz) tomatoes

175 g (6 oz) carrots

1 garlic clove

2.5 cm (1 inch) piece fresh
   horseradish

2–3 ice cubes

Peel and roughly chop the ginger. Trim the celery and cut it into 5 cm (2 inch) lengths. Juice the tomatoes, carrots, garlic and horseradish with the ginger and celery.

Transfer the juice to a food processor or blender, add a couple of ice cubes and process briefly.

Pour the juice into a small glass, garnish with celery slivers, if liked, and serve immediately.

For carrot & pink grapefruit juice
Peel and segment a pink grapefruit, leaving some pith, and juice with 2 carrots and 2 apples. Serve topped up with mineral water.

A spice that packs a punch, GINGER contains gingerol, a powerful anti-inflammatory that may reduce inflammatory pain in the body.

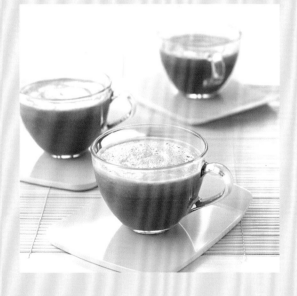

RED REFRESHER JUICE

Serves 1

2 **red peppers**, about 350 g
   (11½ oz) in total

1 lime, plus extra to decorate

½ cucumber, about 175 g (6 oz)

100 g (3½ oz) broccoli

ice cubes

Core and deseed the peppers. Roughly peel the lime. Juice together with the cucumber and broccoli.

Pour the juice into a glass over ice, add slices of lime and serve immediately.

For red hot juice

Core and deseed 2 red peppers – about 350 g (11½ oz) in total. Juice the peppers with 1 small red chilli, 2 carrots – about 300 g (10 oz) in total – and 100 g (3½ oz) broccoli.

RED PEPPERS get their vibrant colour from anthocyanins, natural compounds that may protect brain cells and slow age-related cognitive decline.

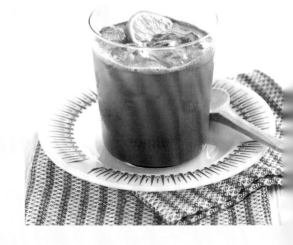

HEALING GREEN JUICE

Serves 2

40 g (1½ oz) **kale**

30 g (1¼ oz) spinach

1 Little Gem lettuce, about
   140 g (4½ oz)

2 celery sticks

½ cucumber, about 175 g (6 oz)

1 apple, about 100 g (3½ oz)

½ teaspoon spirulina powder

1 teaspoon hemp seed oil

ice cubes

Juice the kale with the spinach, lettuce, celery, cucumber and apple. Stir in the spirulina powder and hemp seed oil.

Pour the juice into glasses over ice and serve immediately.

For healing beet juice
Juice 40 g (1½ oz) kale with ½ cucumber – about 175 g (6 oz), 1 beetroot – about 150 g (5 oz), 1 apple – about 100 g (3½ oz) – and a 2 cm (¾ inch) piece peeled fresh root ginger. Stir in ½ teaspoon chlorella powder. Serve poured over ice.

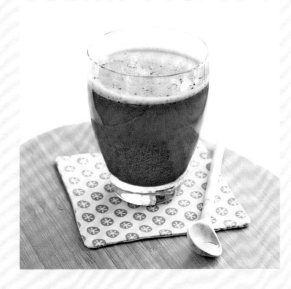

KALE is a plant-based source of calcium, and it also includes vitamin K, which together help strengthen bones.

PINEAPPLE, PARSNIP & CARROT SMOOTHIE

Serves 2

250 g (8 oz) pineapple, plus
    extra to serve (optional)
+ 100 g (3½ oz) **parsnips**
100 g (3½ oz) carrots
75 ml (3 fl oz) soya milk
ice cubes

Peel the pineapple, remove the core and cut the flesh into chunks. Juice the parsnips and carrots with the pineapple.

Transfer the juice to a food processor or blender, add the soya milk and some ice cubes and process until smooth.

Pour the mixture into 2 short glasses, decorate with pineapple wedges, if liked, and serve immediately.

For carrot, orange & banana smoothie
Juice 150 g (5 oz) carrots with 100 g (3½ oz) orange, then blend with 100 g (3½ oz) banana and 6 dried apricots.

Shown to have a calming and sedative effect on the brain, the phytonutrient falcarinol is found in PARSNIPS (and carrots).

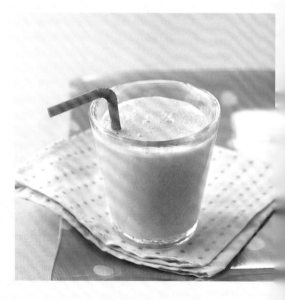

NUTTY RECOVERY SMOOTHIE

Serves 4

4 bananas

4 medjool dates

3 tablespoons **peanut butter**

300 ml (½ pint) almond milk

¼ teaspoon ground cinnamon

Peel the bananas.

Add the bananas to a food processor or blender along with all the remaining ingredients and process until smooth.

Pour the smoothie into 4 glasses and serve immediately.

For kiwi recovery smoothie
Peel and then juice 2 kiwifruit, about 150 g (5 oz). Transfer the juice to a food processor or blender, add the almond milk, cinnamon, 5 dried figs, 1 tablespoon protein powder and 4 walnut halves, omitting the bananas, dates and peanut butter. Process until smooth.

PEANUT BUTTER is a source of protein, a macronutrient essential for building and repairing muscles.

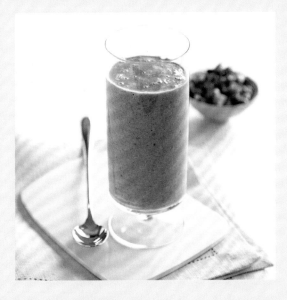

HEALTHY GREEN PUNCH

Serves 1

2 lemons

  1 cm (½ inch) piece fresh
horseradish root
1 apple, about 100 g (3½ oz)
15 g (½ oz) parsley

Roughly peel the lemons. Juice all the ingredients together.

Pour the juice into a glass and serve immediately.

For spicy lemon tea
Juice 2 roughly peeled lemons and a 1 cm (½ inch) piece fresh horseradish root, pour into a cup and top up with boiling water.

HORSERADISH
contains cancer-fighting
compounds known as
glucosinolates, which
activate enzymes
involved in detoxifying
cancer-causing
molecules.

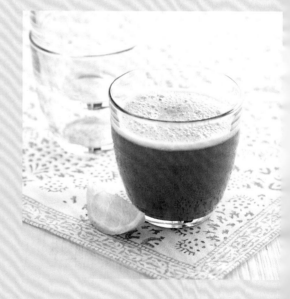

TOMATO, LEMON & PARSLEY JUICE

Serves 1

2 celery sticks, plus leaves
   to serve (optional)
4 tomatoes
large handful of **parsley**
rind and juice of ½ lemon
ice cubes

Trim the celery sticks and cut them into
5 cm (2 inch) lengths. Juice the tomatoes and
parsley with the celery, lemon juice and rind.

Pour the juice into a tall glass over ice, add the
celery leaves, if using, and serve immediately.

For tomato & celery juice
Replace the lemon juice and rind and the
parsley with Tabasco sauce, celery salt and
black pepper, to taste.

**PARSLEY is used as
a natural remedy for
cleansing. It contains
the oil apiol, which is
known for its ability to
support detoxification.**

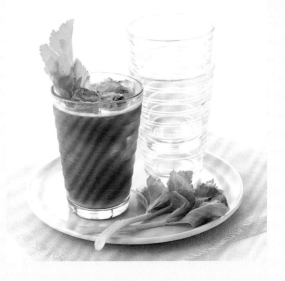

LETTUCE & KIWIFRUIT JUICE

Serves 1

100 g (3½ oz) kiwifruit, plus
    extra to serve (optional)

+ 200 g (7 oz) **lettuce**
    ice cubes (optional)

Peel the kiwifruit and roughly chop the flesh. Separate the lettuce into leaves. Juice the kiwifruit and lettuce, alternating the ingredients so that the lettuce leaves do not clog the machine.

Pour the juice into a glass over ice, if using, decorate with slices of kiwifruit, if liked, and serve immediately.

For lettuce & camomile juice
Juice ½ lemon with 200 g (7 oz) lettuce. Mix the juice with 100 ml (3½ fl oz) chilled camomile tea and serve with a couple of ice cubes and a slice of lemon.

Mildly sedative, lactucin is a bitter milky substance found in LETTUCE known to have a calming effect on the nervous system, which may aid sleep.

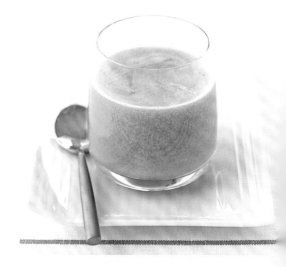

BANANA & MAPLE SYRUP SMOOTHIE

Serves 2

2 bananas

300 ml (½ pint) milk

4 tablespoons natural
   fromage frais

3 tablespoons **maple syrup**

50 g (2 oz) muesli

To decorate

banana slices

malt loaf chunks

Peel and chop the bananas.

Place the bananas in a food processor or blender with the milk, fromage frais and maple syrup and process until smooth. Add the muesli and process again to thicken.

Pour into 2 glasses. Arrange banana slices and chunks of malt loaf on 2 cocktail sticks and balance them across the top of the glasses, to decorate.

For peanut butter smoothies
Replace the bananas with 4 tablespoons crunchy peanut butter and the maple syrup with honey. Make as above.

With a better nutritional profile than white table sugar, MAPLE SYRUP is a healthier alternative.

V

You can swap the dairy milk and fromage frais for any kind of plant-based alternatives.

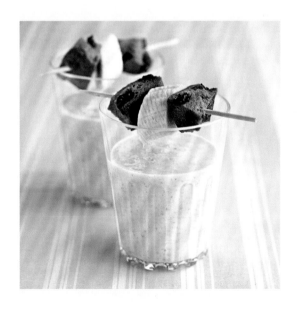

CREAMY PEACH SMOOTHIE

Serves 1

1 large peach

150 ml (¼ pint) natural yogurt

50 ml (2 fl oz) milk

raspberries, to decorate

Skin the peach, remove the stone and roughly chop the flesh. Put the peach, yogurt and milk in a food processor or blender and process until smooth.

Pour the smoothie into a glass, decorate with raspberries and serve immediately.

For pineapple, banana & strawberry smoothie

Juice 100 g (3½ oz) strawberries with 300 g (10 oz) pineapple. Put the juice in a food processor or blender, add a banana and process until smooth.

LIVE YOGURT has probiotics known to benefit gut health by promoting beneficial bacteria growth and improving digestion.

You can swap the dairy milk and yogurt for any kind of plant-based alternatives, such as oat, coconut, soya, etc.

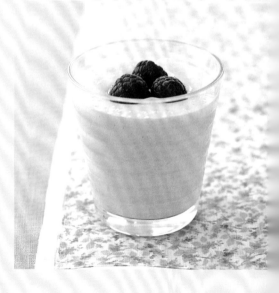

ORANGE & CRANBERRY JUICE

Serves 1

1 orange, about 200 g (7 oz)
225 g (7½ oz) cranberries
2 carrots, about 300 g (10 oz)
  in total

Roughly peel the orange. Juice the orange with the cranberries and carrots.

Pour into a glass and serve immediately.

For cranberry fizz
Juice 225 g (7½ oz) cranberries with 100 g (3½ oz) raspberries and 1 apple – about 100 g (3½ oz). Serve poured over ice and topped up with sparkling water.

Folate plays an important role in supporting a healthy pregnancy, and CITRUS FRUITS are rich in folate, especially oranges.

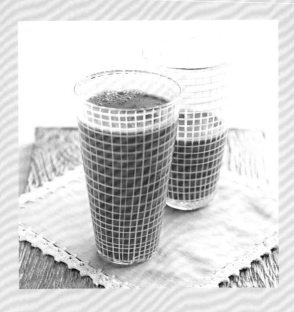

POMEGRANATE PLUS JUICE

Serves 1

+ 1 lemon
+ **2 pomegranates**, about 500 g (1 lb) in total
+ 200 g (7 oz) blueberries

Roughly peel the lemon. Remove the seeds from the pomegranate by cutting the fruit in half, then holding the halved fruit over a bowl and hitting the skin with a wooden spoon so that the seeds fall into the bowl. Juice all the ingredients together.

Pour into a glass and serve immediately.

For peachy pomegranate juice
Remove the seeds from 1 pomegranate – about 250 g (8 oz) in total. Juice the pomegranate seeds with 2 stoned peaches – about 300 g (10 oz) in total, 1 apple – about 100 g (3½ oz) – and 1 carrot – about 150 g (5 oz).

POMEGRANATE JUICE contains an antioxidant called ellagic acid that offers anti-cancer effects, inhibiting prostate cancer cell growth.

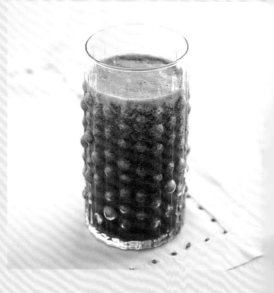

GREEN LEMONADE

Serves 2

2 lemons, plus extra
   to decorate
30 g (1¼ oz) spinach
1 cucumber, about 350 g
   (11½ oz)
sparkling water

Juice the lemons with the spinach
and cucumber.

Pour the juice into glasses, top up with
sparkling water and decorate with a
wedge of lemon.

For citrusade
Replace the spinach with 2 oranges – about
325 g (11 oz) in total – and juice as above.

**This zesty CITRUS
FRUIT is high in natural
citric acid, which
can enhance kidney
function and reduce
the risk of kidney
stone formation.**

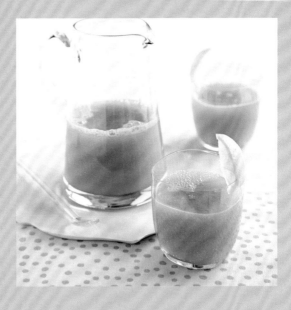

PAPAYA, ORANGE & BANANA SMOOTHIE

Serves 2–3

 1 ripe **papaya**
1 ripe banana
juice of 1 orange
300 ml (½ pint) apple juice
2–3 ice cubes

Process the flesh of a papaya with a banana in a food processor or blender, then add the juice of 1 orange and 300 ml (½ pint) apple juice.

Pour the mixture into 2–3 short glasses and serve immediately.

For banana, mango & orange smoothie
Peel and slice the banana. Instead of papaya, peel 1 ripe mango, remove the stone and roughly chop the flesh. Put the banana, mango 200 ml (7 fl oz) orange juice, 200 ml (7 fl oz) semi-skimmed milk, 3 tablespoons fromage frais and a couple of ice cubes in a food processor or blender and process until smooth

PAPAYA contains the enzyme papain. Together with the fruit's natural fibre, they have been shown to aid digestion, prevent constipation and cleanse the colon.

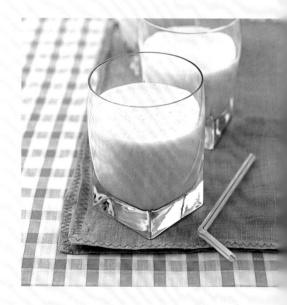

PERFECT PASSION SMOOTHIE

Serves 4

1 lime
2 large mangoes, about 1.15 kg
   (2¼ lb)
5 passion fruit
225 ml (7½ fl oz) natural yogurt
2 handfuls of ice cubes

Roughly peel and then juice the lime. Peel and stone the mangoes.

Transfer the lime juice and mangoes to a food processor or blender. Halve the passion fruit, scoop out the pulp and add all but 1 tablespoon to the blender with the yogurt and ice cubes and process until smooth.

Pour the smoothie into 4 glasses, decorate with the remaining passion fruit pulp and serve immediately.

Piceatannol, a compound found in the seeds of PASSION FRUIT, could improve insulin sensitivity, helping reduce the risk of diseases such as diabetes.

You can also use a plant-based yogurt such as oat, coconut, soya, etc.

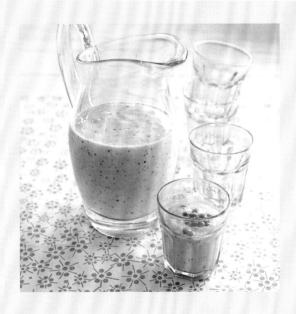

PEAR & PINEAPPLE JUICE

Serves 1

200 g (7 oz) fresh pineapple
   or canned pineapple in
   its own juices
½ lemon
 2 pears
ice cubes

Peel and core the fresh pineapple and cut the flesh into pieces. If using canned pineapple, drain and discard the juice. Juice the lemon with the pineapple and pears.

Pour the juice into a glass over ice and serve immediately.

For pear & kiwifruit juice
Replace both the lemon and pineapple with 3 kiwifruit. This is an excellent juice for all-round good health.

PEARS are high in insoluble fibre, making them a good bulking laxative. This helps the bowels stay regular and supports the good bacteria in the gut.

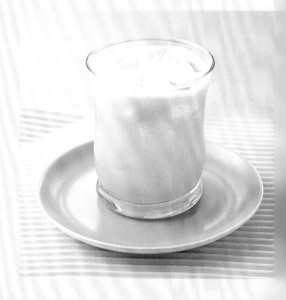

ORANGE, APPLE & PEAR JUICE

Serves 1

2 oranges

1 red apple

1 pear

ice cubes (optional)

1 teaspoon clear honey
(optional)

Peel the oranges and divide the flesh into segments. Chop the apple and pear into even-sized pieces. Juice all the fruit.

Pour the juice into a glass over ice, if using, stir in the honey, if using, and serve immediately.

For apple & pear slush
Roughly chop 2 pears and 2 apples, then process the juice in a food processor or blender with some ice.

An anti-inflammatory compound called nobiletin, found in ORANGES, may help people with inflammatory health conditions by inhibiting pro-inflammatory responses.

Honey can be swapped for maple or agave syrup as a vegan-friendly alternative.

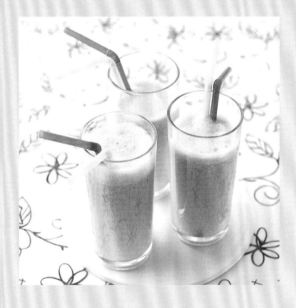

CITRUS GREEN JUICE

Serves 1

1 lime

1 orange, about 200 g (7 oz)

1 grapefruit, about 275 g (9 oz)

1 teaspoon agave syrup

 ½ tablespoon **wheatgrass powder**

Roughly peel the lime, orange and grapefruit. Juice all the fruits together. Stir in the agave syrup and wheatgrass powder.

Pour the juice into a glass and serve immediately.

For gingered green juice
Juice 2 oranges – about 400 g (13 oz) in total, with 2 carrots – about 300 g (10 oz) in total, 1 apple – about 100 g (3½ oz) – and a 2 cm ¾ inch) piece peeled fresh root ginger. Stir in ½ tablespoon barleygrass or wheatgrass powder and serve.

The vibrant green of WHEATGRASS comes from chlorophyll, a natural compound which has therapeutic benefits because of its antioxidant properties.

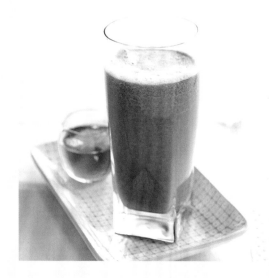

PEACH & ORANGE SMOOTHIE

Serves 2

400 g (13 oz) can **peaches**
   in natural juice
150 ml (¼ pint) natural yogurt,
   plus extra to serve
200 ml (7 fl oz) orange juice
clear honey (optional)
2–3 ice cubes (optional)

Drain the peaches, discarding the juice, and put them in a food processor or blender with the yogurt, orange juice, honey, if using, and a couple of ice cubes, if liked. Process until smooth.

Pour the mixture into 2 short glasses and top with a swirl of any remaining yogurt.

For citrus yogurt smoothie
Put 200 g (7 oz) canned grapefruit in natural juice in a food processor or blender with 150 ml (¼ pint) lemon-flavoured yogurt and 150 ml (¼ pint) semi-skimmed milk. Process until smooth.

PEACHES contain both soluble and insoluble fibre. Soluble fibre helps regulate blood sugar and maintain healthy cholesterol levels.

You can also use a plant-based yogurt. Swap honey for maple or agave syrup as a vegan-friendly alternative.

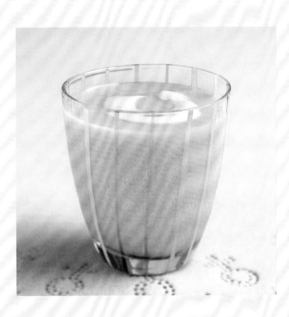

TROPICAL FRUIT SMOOTHIE

Serves 2–3

1 large banana

1 large ripe mango

 150 ml (¼ pint) natural yogurt

300 ml (½ pint) **pineapple juice**

pineapple chunks, to serve (optional)

Peel and slice the banana, then put it in a freezer-proof container and freeze for at least 2 hours or overnight.

Peel the mango, remove the stone and roughly chop the flesh. Place the flesh in a food processor or blender with the frozen banana, yogurt and pineapple juice and process until smooth.

Pour the smoothie into 2–3 tall glasses, decorate with pineapple chunks, if liked, and serve immediately.

PINEAPPLES contain bromelain, an enzyme that has an anti-inflammatory effect stimulating the body to make substances that fight pain and swelling.

V

You can also use a plant-based yogurt such as oat, coconut, soya, etc.

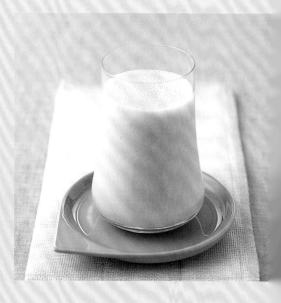

PEACHY PLUM JUICE

Serves 1

4 **plums**, about 300 g (10 oz)
   in total
3 peaches, about 450 g
   (14½ oz) in total
2 apricots, about 150 g
   (5 oz) in total
1 carrot, about 150 g (5 oz)
ice cubes

Remove the stones from the plums, peaches and apricots. Juice all the ingredients together.

Pour the juice into a glass over ice and serve immediately.

For gingered plum juice
Stone 4 plums – about 300 g (10 oz) in total. Juice the plums with 2 carrots – about 300 g (10 oz) in total – and a 2 cm (¾ inch) piece peeled fresh root ginger. Stir in a large pinch of grated nutmeg and serve.

Chlorogenic acid, a polyphenol found in PLUMS, may help regulate blood sugar levels and appetite.

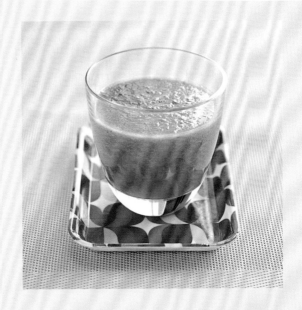

SPINACH, TOMATO & BROCCOLI JUICE

Serves 1

 150 g (5 oz) **spinach**
150 g (5 oz) broccoli
2 tomatoes
celery stick, to serve (optional)

Rinse the spinach and trim the broccoli. Juice the tomatoes with the green vegetables, adding the broccoli and spinach alternately so that the spinach leaves do not clog the juicer.

Pour the juice into a glass, add a stick of celery, if liked, and serve immediately.

For spinach & carrot juice
Rinse 250 g (8 oz) spinach and juice the leaves with 250 g (8 oz) carrots and 25 g (1 oz) parsley. Stir in 1 teaspoon spirulina, the freshwater algae supplement, for extra energy.

Found in SPINACH, lutein and zeaxanthin are carotenoids, a plant-based source of vitamin A, which plays a vital role in maintaining good eye health.

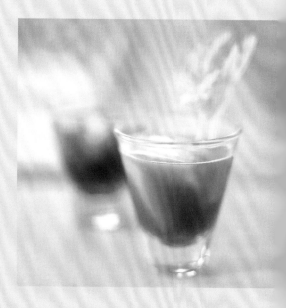

APPLE, PINEAPPLE & MELON JUICE

Serves 1

- galia melon
- **pineapple**
- green apples
- ice cubes (optional)

Peel and deseed the melon. Remove the skin and hard core from the pineapple. Chop all the fruit into even-sized pieces and juice.

Pour the juice into a glass over ice, if using, and serve immediately.

For plum & apple juice
Remove the stones from 5 ripe plums, then juice them with 3 red apples. Serve this delicious juice over ice.

Manganese, a mineral found in PINEAPPLE, may enhance male fertility by improving sperm motility.

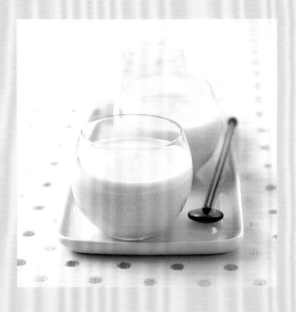

PRUNE, APPLE & CINNAMON SMOOTHIE

Serves 1

+ 65 g (2½ oz) ready-to-eat **prunes**

pinch of ground cinnamon, plus extra to serve

350 ml (12 fl oz) apple juice

❯ 3 tablespoons Greek yogurt

ice cubes

Roughly chop the prunes. Put the prunes and cinnamon in a large bowl, pour over the apple juice, cover and leave to stand overnight.

Put the prunes, apple juice and yogurt in a food processor or blender and process until smooth.

Pour the smoothie into a large glass over ice cubes, sprinkle with extra cinnamon and drink immediately.

For apple & avocado smoothie
Process the flesh of 1 small, ripe avocado with 100 ml (3½ fl oz) apple juice.

Naturally occurring prebiotics in PRUNES promote the growth of beneficial bacteria in your gut, supporting good digestive health.

You can also use a plant-based yogurt such as oat, coconut, soya, etc.

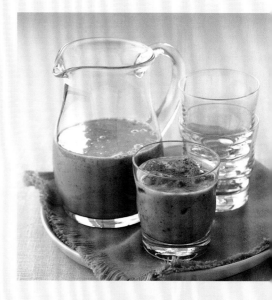

RASPBERRY & BLUEBERRY SMOOTHIE

Serves 1

250 g (8 oz) **raspberries**

200 ml (7 fl oz) apple juice

200 g (7 oz) blueberries

4 tablespoons Greek yogurt

100 ml (3½ fl oz) skimmed milk

1 tablespoon clear honey, or
   to taste

1 tablespoon wheatgerm
   (optional)

Purée the raspberries with half the apple juice. Purée the blueberries with the remaining apple juice.

Mix together the yogurt, milk, honey and wheatgerm, if using, and add a spoonful of the raspberry purée.

Pour the blueberry purée into a tall glass. Carefully pour over the yogurt mixture, and then pour the raspberry purée. Serve chilled.

For vanilla berry juice
Process 150 g (5 oz) frozen mixed berries with 300 ml (½ pint) vanilla-flavoured soya milk and 1 teaspoon clear honey.

RASPBERRIES contain non-haem iron which carries oxygen to all cells, maintaining healthy energy levels.

You can also use a plant-based yogurt or milk and swap honey for maple or agave syrup.

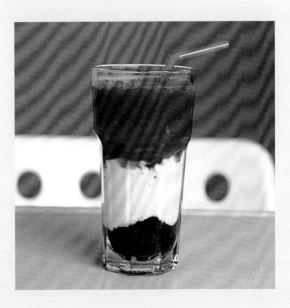

CARROT, RADISH & CUCUMBER JUICE

Serves 1

+ 100 g (3½ oz) potato
100 g (3½ oz) **radish**, plus extra
  to serve (optional)
100 g (3½ oz) carrot
100 g (3½ oz) cucumber
ice cubes

Juice the potato, radish, carrot and cucumber.

Transfer the juice to a food processor or blender, add a couple of ice cubes and process briefly.

Pour the juice into a tall glass over ice, decorate with slices of radish, if liked, and serve immediately.

For carrot, radish & ginger juice
Omit the potato and cucumber and add 2.5 cm (1 inch) peeled and roughly chopped fresh root ginger. This is a good juice if you have a cold or blocked sinuses.

An antifungal protein in RADISH has been found to destroy a common yeast in the body that causes infections like thrush.

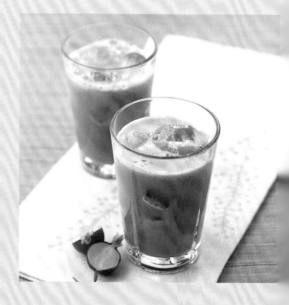

WATERMELON & RASPBERRY JUICE

Serves 1

about 300 g (10 oz) watermelon
125 g (4 oz) **raspberries**
2–3 ice cubes

Skin and deseed the melon and cut the flesh into cubes. Juice the melon with the raspberries.

Pour into a glass, add a couple of ice cubes and serve immediately.

For watermelon & orange juice
Juice 2 oranges instead of the raspberries.

Initial research has found that rheosmin (RASPBERRY KETONES) might suppress appetite and stimulate metabolism, potentially helping with weight loss.

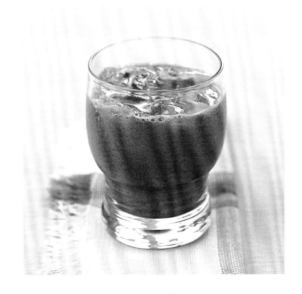

CARROT, CABBAGE & APPLE JUICE

Serves 1

175 g (6 oz) carrots
250 g (8 oz) apples
125 g (4 oz) **red cabbage**
orange slices, to decorate
ice cubes

Roughly chop the carrots and apples and juice them with the cabbage.

Pour the juice into a glass over ice, decorate with a slice of orange, and serve immediately.

For carrot, spinach & pink grapefruit juice
Juice 125 g (4 oz) each of carrot, spinach and pink grapefruit. This juice has a pleasantly astringent flavour.

CABBAGE and other cruciferous vegetables contain sulphoraphane, an antioxidant that may lower the risk of heart disease by reducing inflammation.

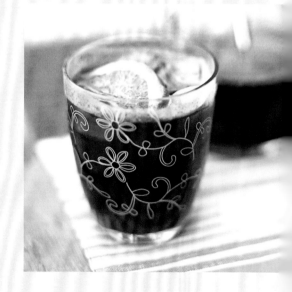

RHUBARB SMOOTHIE

Serves 2

100 g (3½ oz) stewed **rhubarb**

100 ml (3½ fl oz) natural yogurt

2 drops vanilla extract

honey, to taste

Blend the stewed rhubarb with the yogurt and vanilla extract. Sweeten to taste with honey.

Pour the mixture into 2 short glasses over ice, if using, and serve immediately.

For choco-cherry shake
Blend 100 g (3½ oz) pitted cherries with 100 ml (3½ fl oz) soya milk and 25 g (1 oz) melted dark chocolate. Serve with ice.

RHUBARB contains sennosides (also found in senna), which act as natural laxatives and help promote healthy bowel movements.

Honey can be swapped for maple or agave syrup as a vegan-friendly alternative.

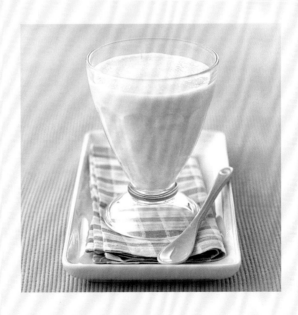

ORANGE, MANGO & STRAWBERRY SMOOTHIE

Serves 2

125 g (4 oz) **strawberries**
1 small ripe mango
300 ml (½ pint) orange juice
orange slices, to decorate
    (optional)

Hull the strawberries, put them in a freezer container and freeze for 2 hours or overnight.

Peel the mango, remove the stone, roughly chop the flesh and put it in a food processor or blender with the strawberries and orange juice and process until thick.

Pour the smoothie into 2 tall glasses, decorate with slices of orange, if liked, and serve immediately.

For orange & banana smoothie
Blend 1 ripe banana with the strawberries and orange juice. Serve decorated with orange slices, if liked.

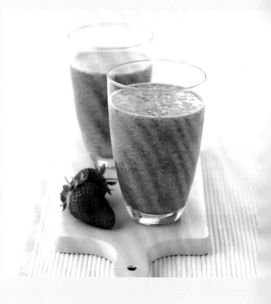

Bright red and glossy, these juicy STRAWBERRIES are rich in vitamin C, which helps the body to absorb energy-boosting iron.

PURPLE POWER JUICE

Serves 1

2 cm (¾ inch) piece fresh
   root ginger
100 g (3½ oz) red cabbage
1 celery stick
1 apple, about 100 g (3½ oz)
12 red grapes
ice cubes

Peel the ginger. Juice together the peeled ginger, cabbage, celery, apple and grapes.

Pour the juice into a glass over ice and serve immediately.

For purple protein juice
Juice 100 g (3½ oz) red cabbage with 12 red grapes, 1 beetroot – about 125 g (4 oz) – and 2 carrots – about 300 g (10 oz) in total. Whisk in 1 tablespoon protein powder and serve.

Resveratrol is a stilbenoid from RED GRAPES that possesses strong antioxidant activity and has been shown to have anti-cancer activity.

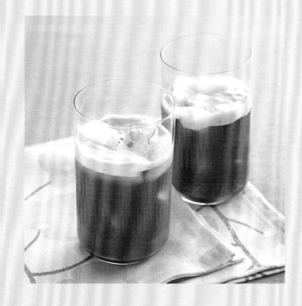

TOMATO, RED PEPPER & PAPAYA JUICE

Serves 1

about 125 g (4 oz) papaya

about 100 g (3½ oz) red
 pepper

 1 large **tomato**

2–3 ice cubes

Peel and deseed the papaya. Core and deseed the pepper. Juice the tomato with the papaya and pepper.

Transfer the juice to a food processor or blender, add a couple of ice cubes and process together.

Pour into a glass and serve immediately.

For pepper & orange juice
Core and deseed 100 g (3½ oz) each of red, yellow and orange peppers and juice the pepper flesh with 1 orange. Serve sprinkled with chopped mint.

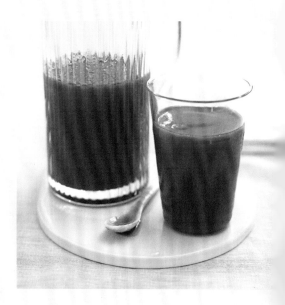

TOMATOES are rich in the carotenoid pigment lycopene, which has been found to affect bone density and help retain bone strength.

CARROT, BEETROOT & SWEET POTATO JUICE

Serves 1

175 g (6 oz) **sweet potato**

100 g (3½ oz) beetroot

175 g (6 oz) carrots

125 g (4 oz) fennel

ice cubes

fennel fronds, to decorate
   (optional)

Peel the sweet potato and scrub the beetroot. Juice the carrots and fennel with the sweet potato and beetroot.

Pour into a glass over ice, decorate with fennel fronds, if liked, and serve immediately.

For carrot, beetroot & orange juice
Replace the sweet potato and fennel with 125 g (4 oz) strawberries and 1 orange. This colourful juice will give you an instant energy boost.

Useful for glucose control, SWEET POTATOES contain the hormone adiponectin, which, together with slow-release carbohydrates, keeps blood sugars low.

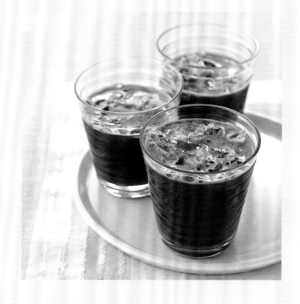

ENERGIZER SMOOTHIE

Serves 2

1 beetroot, about 200 g (7 oz)

6 dates, stoned

✚ 1 tablespoon **rolled oats**

100 g (3½ oz) blackberries

1 teaspoon maca powder

500 ml (17 fl oz) almond milk

1 teaspoon ground flaxseed

ice cubes

Juice the beetroot.

Transfer the juice to a food processor or blender, add the remaining ingredients (except the ice cubes) and process until smooth.

Pour the smoothie into 2 glasses over ice and serve immediately.

For spicy energizer smoothie
Juice 1 beetroot with a 3 cm (1¼ inch) piece peeled fresh root ginger and 1 lemon grass stalk. Blend in a food processor with 6 figs, 1 tablespoon rolled oats, 100 g (3½ oz) strawberries, 1 teaspoon maca powder and 500 ml (17 fl oz) almond milk until smooth.

ROLLED OATS are a great source of beta-glucan, a soluble fibre that supports the gut by feeding the good bacteria that live there.

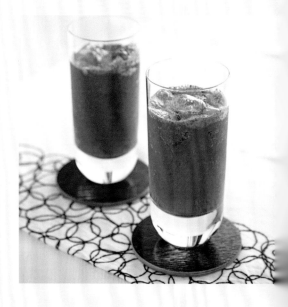

WATERMELON COOLER

Serves 2

100 g (3½ oz) **watermelon**

100 g (3½ oz) strawberries

100 ml (3½ fl oz) still water

small handful of mint or
   tarragon leaves, plus extra
   to serve (optional)

Skin and deseed the melon and chop the flesh into cubes. Hull the strawberries. Freeze the melon and strawberries until solid.

Put the frozen melon and strawberries in a food processor or blender, add the water and the mint or tarragon and process until smooth.

Pour the mixture into 2 short glasses, decorate with mint or tarragon leaves, if liked, and serve immediately.

For melon & almond smoothie
Process 100 g (3½ oz) frozen galia melon flesh with 100 ml (3½ fl oz) almond milk.

WATERMELONS are a rich source of the plant pigment lycopene, which has been shown to protect cells from damage, decreasing cancer risk.

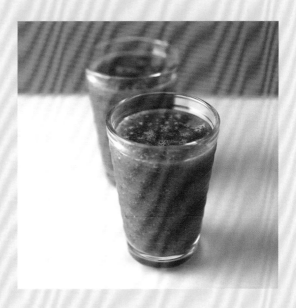

WATERCRESS & PEPPER PUNCH

Serves 2

1 red pepper, about 175 g (6 oz)

1 beetroot, about 125 g (4 oz)

2 carrots, about 300 g (10 oz)
   in total

½ lemon

 50 g (2 oz) **watercress**

ice cubes

pepper, to sprinkle

Core and deseed the red pepper. Juice together with the beetroot, carrots, lemon and watercress.

Pour the juice into 2 glasses over ice, sprinkle with black pepper and serve immediately.

For hot pepper punch
Core and deseed 1 red pepper – about 175 g (6 oz). Juice the pepper with 2 celery sticks, 3 tomatoes – about 300 g (10 oz) in total, 2 carrots – about 300 g (10 oz) in total – and a 2 cm (¾ inch) piece fresh horseradish root.

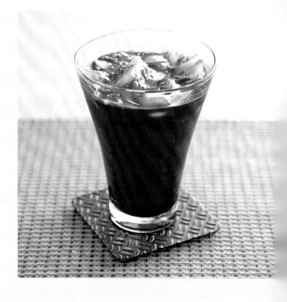

WATERCRESS is known to have blood-cleansing properties due the presence of sulphur-containing glucosinolates.

TOMATO, ORANGE & CELERY JUICE

Serves 2

2 oranges

2 celery sticks, plus leafy
  stalks to serve

4 tomatoes

2 carrots

ice cubes

Peel the oranges. Trim the celery and cut it into 5 cm (2 inch) lengths. Juice the tomatoes and carrots with the oranges and celery.

Pour the juice into 2 tall glasses over ice, decorate with leafy celery stick stirrers and serve immediately.

For celery & apple juice
Trim and cut 3 celery sticks into 5 cm (2 inch) lengths. Juice the celery with 2 apples and 25 g (1 oz) alfalfa sprouts.

Lipoic acid, an antioxidant found in TOMATOES, has been shown to reduce insulin resistance and improve blood sugar control.

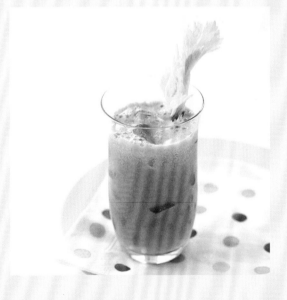

STRAWBERRY, REDCURRANT & ORANGE JUICE

Serves 1

100 g (3½ oz) strawberries

75 g (3 oz) **redcurrants**, plus extra to serve (optional)

½ orange

125 ml (4 fl oz) still water

½ teaspoon clear honey (optional)

ice cubes

Hull the strawberries. Remove the stalks from the redcurrants and peel and segment the orange. Juice the fruit, add the water and stir in the honey, if using.

Pour the juice into a glass, add some ice cubes and decorate with extra redcurrants, if liked. To make this juice into lollies, pour into lolly moulds after stirring in the honey and freeze.

For kiwifruit & orange juice
Roughly chop 3 kiwifruit and juice with 2 large oranges.

REDCURRANTS are rich in vitamin C, which supports the immune system, reducing the risk of viral and bacterial infections.

V

Honey can be swapped for maple or agave syrup as a vegan-friendly alternative.

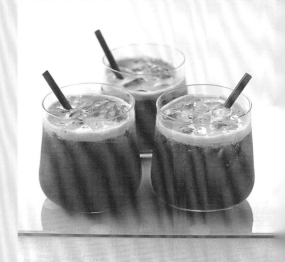

STRAWBERRY & SOYA SMOOTHIE

Serves 1

100 g (3½ oz) fresh or frozen
   strawberries
200 ml (7 fl oz) **soya milk**
2 kiwifruit
ice cubes (optional)
25 g (1 oz) flaked almonds,
   to decorate (optional)

Hull the strawberries. Put them into a food processor or blender with the soya milk and kiwifruit and process briefly. If you are using fresh rather than frozen strawberries, add a few ice cubes, if using, and process until smooth.

Pour into a glass, decorate with flaked almonds, if liked, and serve immediately.

For summer berry & honey smoothie
Put 125 g (4 oz) frozen mixed berries into a food processor or blender with 300 ml (½ pint) grape juice, 3 tablespoons quark and 1 teaspoon clear honey. Process until smooth.

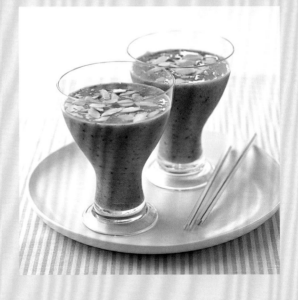

SOYA MILK is a natural source of phytoestrogens, which mimic the hormone oestrogen, helping to alleviate peri-menopausal symptoms.

BANANA & TAHINI SMOOTHIE

Serves 1–2

1 ripe banana

 300 ml (½ pint) semi-skimmed milk

2 teaspoons **tahini paste**

Peel and slice the banana, put it in a freezer container and freeze for at least 2 hours or overnight.

Put the banana, milk and tahini paste in a food processor or blender and process until smooth.

Pour the smoothie into 1–2 tall glasses and serve immediately.

For banana almond smoothie

Put 2 frozen bananas, 450 ml (¾ pint) soya milk, 40 g (1½ oz) ground almonds and a pinch of cinnamon into a food processor or blender and process briefly.

TAHINI is made from sesame seeds, a plant-based source of calcium, which is needed to build and maintain strong bones.

Swap dairy milk for any kind of plant-based milk, such as oat, coconut (see below), soya, etc.

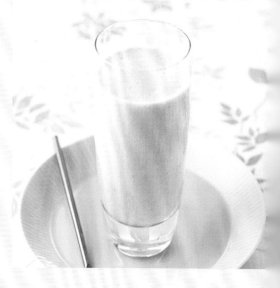

CARROT, PARSNIP & SWEET POTATO JUICE

Serves 1

175 g (6 oz) celery

175 g (6 oz) carrots

175 g (6 oz) parsnips

175 g (6 oz) **sweet potatoes**

handful of parsley, plus an
extra sprig to decorate
(optional)

1 garlic clove

2–3 ice cubes

lemon wedge

Trim the celery and cut it into 5 cm (2 inch) lengths. Juice the carrots, parsnips, sweet potatoes, parsley and garlic with the celery.

Transfer the juice to a food processor or blender and process with the ice cubes.

Pour the juice into a glass, decorate with a wedge of lemon and a parsley sprig, if liked, and serve immediately.

For carrot, parsnip & melon juice
Juice 125 g (4 oz) each of carrots, parsnips, lettuce and cantaloupe melon for a juice that is especially rich in folic acid.

SWEET POTATOES contain beta-carotene and vitamin C, a combination that helps regulate the immune system and enhances the body's natural protection against infections.

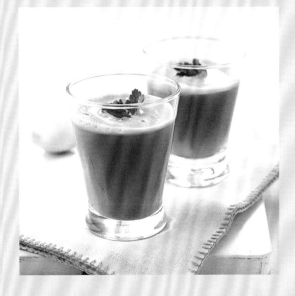

INDEX

GLOSSARY

Beetroot..................................... Beet
Celeriac .... Celery root
Chicory .... Endive
Coriander (fresh)...................... Cilantro
Flaked almonds......................... Slivered almonds
Jug .... Pitcher
Kitchen paper .... Paper towel
Muslin cloth............................... Cheesecloth
Natural yogurt........................... Plain yogurt
Pepper .... Bell pepper
Spring onion.............................. Scallion

ABOUT THE AUTHOR

Nicola Deschamps is a nutritionist, author and editor. Registered with the Association for Nutrition, Nicola has a Master's degree in nutrition, physical activity and public health, and a diploma in nutritional therapy. Nicola writes and edits books on nutrition, health and wellbeing.